Fat Loss Forever

Healthy Andy

DISCLAIMER

The information in this book is no way intended to replace the knowledge or consultation of your personal health provider.

Before you start any diet or exercise program you should consult your physician.

CONTENTS

SECTION 3: GO!!!

Introduction:
On Your Mark...

First off, let me make something clear. I wasn't always "Healthy Andy". In fact, although I was always active and athletic, I've also always struggled with my weight.

Oh, I was never obese, but I definitely carried too much chubb on my belly. And, at one point, it got pretty bad… I was probably thirty pounds overweight or so.

I could feel my abs underneath that pudge, but couldn't seem to get them to come out and play, no matter how hard I tried. My running joke was that I had a six-pack… well, more like "half a case" (I would gesture towards my love handles as I said this).

You might be in the same boat. If you are, let me tell you, I understand your frustration. You may have been trying so hard you want to scream, but the results just aren't there. I hear you. I was right there, pulling my hair out (well, until I started shaving my head) with frustration from not being able to get the body that I wanted.

At one point, I gave up. Oh, it's just genetics, I said. I'm screwed. Can't do anything about it. Gonna just be soft in the belly forever.

Folks, that's a lie. A lie we tell ourselves to let us off the hook of finding a solution to our problems. And once I stopped telling myself that lie, I developed a method to get myself into shape and stay that way.

You can do it too. Hey, if a recovering carb-and-junk-food junkie like me can drop thirty pounds and go from Buddha Belly to Healthy Andy, so can you. It's not magic. There's no voodoo.

The very first thing to do is to realize that you, yes, **YOU**, really can do this. This book will be your guide down the path to the kind of body you've always wanted. And we're going to get there the healthy way… no crazy diet pills or crash dieting or stupidity like that.

Like any other journey, **the first step is to make up your mind** to actually **TAKE** the journey. Then, it's just a matter of plotting a course… and walking the path.

There's something else I want to say. If you've been feeling frustrated, angry, unattractive, or any of those other unpleasant emotions when it comes to your weight… good.

I mean it. Good! I'm not trying to be cruel, it's just that human beings typically only change their behavior due to the **presence of pain**… so let those painful emotions inspire you to finally head off down the road to getting into the kind of shape you want to be in. If you're too content with where you are, you'll never leave. **Being dissatisfied with your current situation is what makes us head for the door**.

Just don't let those negative emotions get out of hand and fool you into thinking nothing will ever change. That's just lies we tell ourselves when we're tired and want an excuse to give up and go back to what we're used to… what we're comfortable with.

We'll talk more about this later. In fact, that's one of the things that sets this book apart from all the other fitness books out there… we're going to go over the **REALLY** difficult stuff: the **MENTAL** part of it. How exactly **DO** you make a lasting fundamental change in your fitness habits to achieve your goals? Especially without making yourself miserable in the process?

WHAT SETS THIS BOOK APART

That's the real "secret" to getting into the kind of super-duper shape that will make all of your friends jealous (and admit it, you want that). So much of the path to fitness is mental, and nobody seems to talk about it.

Seriously! Everybody wants to talk about the specifics of diet and exercise and leave it at that. Make no mistake, the fundamentals of diet and exercise ARE important, obviously… but the truth is, I can cover the principles of what you need to know about diet and exercise in just a few chapters (in fact, that's exactly what I do in this book).

The real task is in incorporating those diet and exercise habits into your life for the long term. And unfortunately, every other weight loss book out there just skips over that part… or shrugs it off with a little "Hey, just stick with it, slugger. Use your willpower."

As you'll see in the section on The Mental Game, that's a bunch of nonsense. Willpower is a myth. It really is. You'll read all about what willpower REALLY is, and why you REALLY can't rely on it for anything. Relying on willpower is what leads to 98% of people failing to keep weight off in the long term.

I don't want that for you. I don't want you to kill yourself with some bizarre crash diet or draconian exercise regime that you can't possibly keep up with in the long term. That just leads to so-called "yo-yo" dieting: lose the weight, gain it back, repeat.

Instead, let me teach you the psychological and physiological keys to changing your habits in the right direction… and keeping it that way for good.

So now you have a choice. Stay where you are, sitting on your couch, wearing your "fat jeans" and eating too many cookies, looking at magazine pictures of beautiful people with beautiful abs, getting angry, getting jealous, wondering why that can't be you.

Or, you can make a change in your life, and get on the road to **BEING** the person in the picture, the one everybody **ELSE** is jealous of.

You can do this. **YOU CAN DO THIS**. Just read this guide, and walk the path.

Okay. Enough intro and pep-talk. I know you're chomping
at the bit and gung-ho to get started. Just remember… the
race to fitness is a marathon, not a sprint. In fact, it's more of
a lifestyle than a race… a race implies a "finish". Forget those
notions. To keep your healthy body once you have it (here's
something nobody else wants to tell you), will require a
lifestyle change that is permanent.

Don't let that intimidate you. We're going to go over how to
make that easy. After all, you already **HAVE** a permanent
lifestyle… it's just that right now, it's for fatness, not fitness.
We're about to change all of that.

You might even enjoy it! I did!

 If you find this book helpful, head on over to the website at

www.healthyandy.com

for more. What kind of more? Nutritional supplements,
articles, podcasts, books, coupons, all kind of good stuff. I'm
also on Facebook and Twitter under the name "Healthy
Andy", where I post whatever health tips and interesting stuff
I find.

Section Two: Get Set (The Mental Game)...

Chapter 1:
The Anatomy of A habit

Here's the most important part of this book. Oh, I know, you thought it was the diet tips, or the ab exercises, right? Nope.

Although knowing what to do is important, **actually following through on those actions and keeping consistent with those actions is far more important**. A wise man once said, "We are what we repetitively do. Excellence, then, is not an event, but a habit".

That wise man's name was Aristotle. Over two thousand years ago, he laid out the truth… We are what our habits are. That simple.

So, if you want to get in great shape, and even better, KEEP in great shape, you're going to need to form and keep the habits that create that in your life. The actions you need to take to get into great shape aren't difficult or complicated.

The question is, will you make them last? Will you make them a habit? The term getting kicked around is **lifestyle modification,** and it's the tricky part of losing fat forever that no other personal trainers or weight-loss gurus want to talk about.

The body has a short memory, my friends. Lose all that fat today, but give up on the diet and exercise habits that got you there, and say goodbye to those six-pack abs. You'll gain all that fat right back, maybe with interest accrued.

Some people moan and groan over that. *I don't wanna have to change*, they cry. You know what? Too bad. That's the way it works. So you can cry about it, or work with it.

That last paragraph is what I sound like when I'm giving out tough love, by the way.

Working with the body, as it turns out, isn't that bad, if you know how to do it right. It simply means learning how to form habits for a lifetime, so you don't give up on your new diet and exercise routines.

Keep the fitness habits, and you keep your fit body. Lose those habits, and that fit body gets fat in no time flat.

I keep hammering on this point because it is CRITICAL. All of those personal trainers and weight loss gurus are failing you when they fail to teach you how to make fitness a habit. They fail you when they just shrug and say "Just stick to it". "Just use your willpower".

Fail. They fail you, because they guarantee you will fail.

Willpower fails. It always fails, **because it's a myth**. In the coming chapters, we're going to explode the myth of willpower and expose it for what it really is (which is quite mundane and boring, actually… you'll see).

You can't rely on willpower. You have to learn how to make fitness a habit, a part of you as natural and easy as walking or riding a bike (assuming you know how to ride a bike!).

What I'm about to show you will set you apart from those 98% of people who will try to lose weight and end up failing. That's a real percentage, by the way. Only 2% of people lose the weight and keep it off with a "regular" weight loss program.

You're going to succeed where they failed, because I'm going to teach you things no other trainer or coach or guru has ever taught you… how to make it last.

Since we're talking about how to build a habit, first we have to look at what makes up a habit. Essentially, we're starting with the anatomy of a habit.

In order to do that, we need to look under the metaphorical hood of a habit and see how it works. What really is a habit? What makes it up? What rules apply to habits?

We'll start by recognizing that a habit is a **psychological** phenomenon, and therefore, is **neurological** in basis. Once we understand the neurology of a habit, we can realize the rules of how they work and make those rules work for us.

Now, some of you might be intimidated by the subject of neurology, or might think it'll be too boring. But the concepts we'll be dealing with are really quite simple. Here's a preview:

- **Neural networks are patterns made up of individual units called *neurons* strung together.**
- **The more neurons, the more complex and powerful the pattern.**
- **The patterns have a specific input which gets the whole thing moving.**

Before we get into it, let's take a step back and look at some ancient wisdom from a fellow named Miyamoto Musashi.

This is where you say, *"Who?"* Trust me on this one.

Miyamoto Musashi was a swordsman in 17th century Japan… perhaps the greatest swordsman who ever lived. Throughout his life, he won duels against something like sixty opponents and fought his way out of situations sometimes pitting he alone against many foes.

In those days, duels were decided at the end of a four-foot long razor blade called a *katana*, or samurai sword as we know it. Towards the end of his life, he reflected on how and why he was able to overcome his adversaries in all situations, and came to realize certain principles of success.

In his book, *The Book Of Five Rings*, Musashi repeatedly uses this phrase… "From one thing, learn ten thousand things".

This phrase has meaning on several levels. For example, in the context of swordplay and combat, which forms the basis of Musashi's book, he stresses that one-on-one combat is no different than ten-on-ten combat; the actions and tactics of armies are essentially the same, in principle, as those of single-combat duelists.

The particular weapons of the combatants were relatively unimportant, either; fighting indoors with short swords worked on the same principles as fighting with spears or long swords outdoors… only the details changed.

But it goes further than that. Musashi's winning principles brought him success in *all* endeavors, martial or otherwise. After retiring to a mountain retreat to meditate, he taught himself to become an accomplished painter… with no master to instruct him.

What Musashi had learned as a swordsman, he applied to the art of painting, and found success there as well. He goes on to relate how he was now free to master anything possible… from one thing, he had learned ten thousand things.

Similarly, we will learn principles of the natural laws of our body and apply them to many areas of weight loss. From one thing, we will learn ten thousand things. Let's begin.

THE STRUCTURE OF A HABIT

Here is the first core concept of this section. The central nervous system (CNS)… which is the brain and spinal cord… runs the whole show. You can think of it as the Master Computer of the body; it makes your muscles move, your lungs breathe, your heart beat, and coordinates millions of chemical reactions in your body at any particular time.

It is also where thought, emotion, and personality all originate. Our skills, memories, reflexes, and creative thoughts reside in the CNS. It isn't inaccurate to state that we are our nervous system, and it is us.

For many years, it was believed that the nervous system was very static; that is, the nerve cells you were born with were essentially the nerve cells you die with. Damage the nervous system, destroy brain cells, and you're out of luck. The circuitry of the CNS, which we'll discuss in a moment, was rigid and inflexible.

The latest in research shoots all kinds of holes in that theory. The cutting edge of neurology centers on neural *plasticity*, which is the ability of the nervous system to shift and mold itself to whatever is necessary for the body. We'll talk about that as well.

For now, I just want you to keep in the forefront of your mind that the CNS, the Master System, is the Big Kahuna when it comes to the body. Nothing else comes close. In fact, you could even make an argument that our bodies are merely a life support system for our central nervous system.

So let's talk a little about the CNS. Don't worry, I promise I won't blow you away with a lot of fancy talk designed to confuse or dazzle you. The basic concepts that we're working with are really quite simple: in fact, as I mentioned in the Introduction, most of you are already aware of them. We'll just explore how they work, so that we can figure out how best to use them.

We'll begin with the most basic unit of the nervous system. Seems like a good starting point, right? Now, I will have to teach you one term, but it's an easy one, and it's the name for the smallest unit of the CNS… the *neuron*. If your CNS is a house, the neuron is a brick.

Okay, great, you say, but what exactly is it? We know its name, but what does is look like, what does it do? Well, it looks a little like this, anatomically (by the way, feel free to be completely dazzled by my artistic skills):

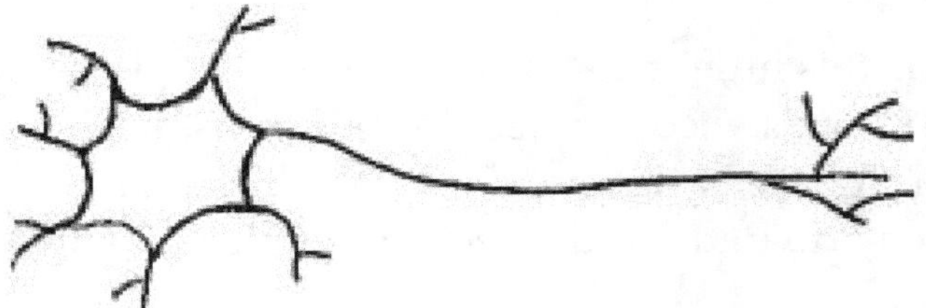

Functionally, it would look a little more like this:

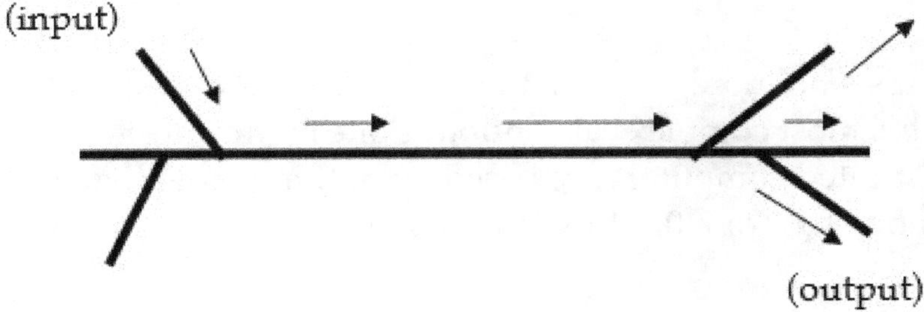

So what are we looking at? Basically, that big bulby thing is the neuron's **cell body**, which is what keeps the neuron alive. If the neuron is like the Pony Express, sending a message along its length, the cell body is the stable where the horses are kept and fed and watered.

Before that (on the left) are the branchy do-dads called *dendrites*… feel free to forget this term, since it's not important to us… and that's where the information comes in.

There can be a lot of these branches (as many as 100,000!) each connecting with a different neuron.

The tail sticking off of the other side is an *axon*… feel free to forget that term also… which is the output, where the information gets sent. It goes off and plugs into another neuron's dendrite (branchy input site).

So what is this little critter's job? In essence, the neuron's sole purpose for existence is to receive and transmit signals; electrical signals, basically. That's it. The signal comes in at the branchy do-dads, and travels down the tail part to the next neuron.

That's it? you say, disbelief in your voice. *You told us this was the most important part of the body, and all it is, is a glorified electrical wire?*

Well, it's a bit more complex than that. But keep in mind that all of the most complex calculations done by the most sophisticated computers are based on nothing more than a variation of a 1 or a 0… binary code.

And essentially, neurons do the same, except it's either "fire" or "not fire". If it sounds impossible that we can create complex patterns and interactions with something so simple, think about what we can do with lights. Lights are either on, or off, right? Fire or not fire, 0 or 1.

Have you ever seen a string of Christmas lights blink in such a way as to give the illusion of the lights "moving"? We've all seen those narrow message boards made up of red lights, which appear to have words "moving" across their surface… usually to tell me my plane has been delayed. Those words, and that movement, are an illusion created by a pattern of nothing more than a bunch of lights either on or not on, firing or not firing, 0 or 1.

The power comes from the pattern, the network. So let's take a look at how the lowly little neuron starts to pick up a little kick.

THE NEURAL NETWORK

In the Internet age, we all know that "networking" increases our computing power dramatically. Now we'll see that same concept at work in our own master computer, the CNS. We'll start with the simplest network, or pattern of neurons hooked together, that I know of: the **simple reflex**.

An example of the simple reflex that we're all familiar with is the knee jerk reflex: you know, that's the one where the doctor whacks you just below the kneecap with his little rubber tomahawk and your leg twitches. Here's a simple diagram, of two neurons linked together to create this action:

THE SIMPLE REFLEX

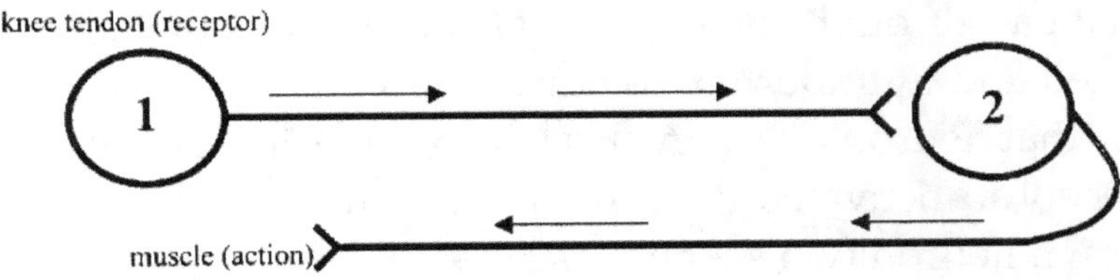

What are we looking at, here? First off, there are little structures in the tendon of the kneecap called *stretch*

receptors, which are exactly what they sound like: they sense when the tendon is being stretched.

When that happens, they send an electrical signal to the branchy end of the first neuron, which starts the whole shebang off. This is actually an important concept to understand for later on. Remember, from one thing, learn ten thousand things? Just keep in mind that all of our neurological patterns are activated by a specific kind of input. Heating up your knee tendon won't activate the knee-jerk reflex, and cold won't, either. Only a stretch… a rapid stretch.

The detailed mechanism of how this works is kind of cool, but it's also complicated and completely unnecessary to our discussion here. Just remember that it's only a specific input that will start off the show. We'll apply this knowledge later when we start dealing with more complex patterns of neural networks.

But back to the basics for now. First, the stretch receptors go *Bing!* and start off an electrical impulse that travels down the length of neuron number one. The tail end of neuron number one then intersects with neuron number two.

There's actually a little gap there, between the end of neuron one and the beginning of neuron two, and the electrical signal jumps that gap through some chemical shenanigans that are complicated and unimportant to our discussion. Just recognize that neuron one activates neuron two, just as the stretch receptors activated neuron one, and an electrical signal shoots down neuron two's length as a result.

Then, as the signal reaches the end of neuron two, we see that a muscle is stuck onto the end of neuron two's tail. The electrical signal jumps that gap, as well, and makes the muscle twitch. In a nutshell, that's a simple reflex. Two neurons, connected together, forming an incredibly simple network, bridging the stretch receptors to the leg muscles.

I like to think of it as a game of Whisper Down the Alley, and the neurons are like kids talking from house to house using a Styrofoam cup and string.

HOWEVER… it's really not quite that simple. Shocking, right? There's actually a little more going on to this simple little network, that makes it look more like this:

THE NOT SO SIMPLE REFLEX

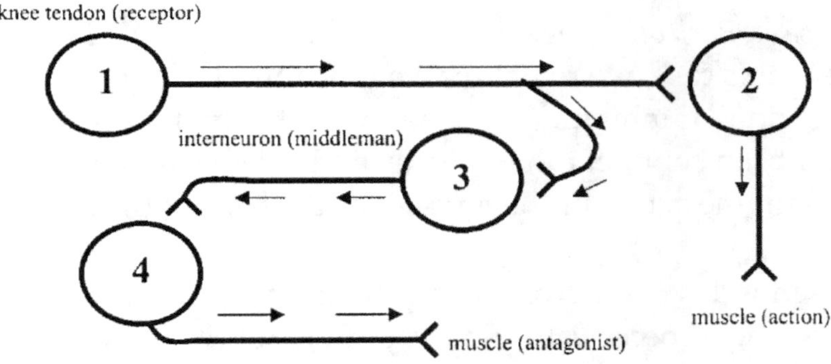

Right. So what's going on NOW? Well, the same thing as before, with a little extra added in. First we see our trusty dusty stretch receptors, getting stretched and excited and firing off that initial electrical impulse.

But this time, not only does neuron one connect with neuron two (which goes to the twitching muscle), it ALSO fires off neuron #3, something called an *interneuron*. Yes, you can forget that term right away; it just means it's a middleman neuron, who shuffles the signal around and decides what other neurons get to be fired off.

It's sort of like that person you call to invite a whole bunch of other people to your party; you don't have all of their phone numbers, so you call that middleman person to invite everybody for you.

In this case, the middleman neuron goes along and invites neuron number four to the party, once again by sending an electrical signal that jumps the gap between them and so on and so forth. The signal shoots down neuron number four, which attaches to the muscles in the back of the leg.

Eh? you say. *Back of the leg? Why the back of the leg?* Well, because in this case, we're not making the muscle twitch… we're relaxing, or inhibiting, it. That way, the thigh muscles in the front can contract more quickly and forcibly and not have to fight the action of the muscles of the back of the leg.

Since the muscles in the front of the leg kick your leg like you're kicking a soccer ball, and the muscles of the back of your leg do the opposite and kick back like you're trying to kick yourself in the butt, if you want one to kick extra hard, you need to make sure the other side isn't tightened up to slow your kick down. So neuron number three shuts the opposite side's muscles down.

Don't let this confuse you. If you need a ride home from work, and it's either Aunt Tilly or Uncle Pete who can do it, once you decide you want Uncle Pete to pick you up, you have to make two phone calls, don't you? One to Uncle Pete to tell him to pick you up, and a second to Aunt Tilly to tell her NOT to pick you up. The first is an action, the second is essentially inhibiting the opposite action. See?

Now our network is a little more complex (four neurons instead of two), and a little more powerful (enhanced twitch speed and power from the opposing muscles being shut down).   And it actually is even more complex than I've illustrated.

In the real simple reflex, middleman neurons go all over the place in your spine when the network is activated, to do everything from make that muscle twitch, to inhibit its opposite, to enhance your balance.

Some middlemen even send signals up to the brain to make sure the twitching isn't too intense and doesn't last too long. This is called *modulation* and is actually a very important concept we'll take a moment to talk about, as it will become important later in the context of willpower and stress.

MODULATE ME!

Okay, so what's the deal with modulation, which I claim is so important? Why are we wasting valuable resources (e.g., extra neurons) with it? Can't we just twitch away, and the heck with the consequences?

Gee, I hope not, because modulation is what keeps you from kicking hard enough to plant your foot in my groin when I elicit the knee-jerk reflex from you in my office. You see, our wonderfully complex brains have developed the ability to end-run our neurological reflexes when the situation is inappropriate.

This is why the doctor tells you to close your eyes when he's planning on whacking your knee with his rubber tomahawk. If you see him doing it, your brain recognizes that your knee isn't *really* getting stretched, and you don't *really* need to contract your leg muscles to keep from falling over, so your noggin cuts off the pattern from ever firing (through a couple of middleman connections like the type we talked about earlier).

The same mechanism, modulation by your higher brain centers, is what keeps the contraction from becoming too intense or lasting too long. If I whack your knee, and keep the hammer pressed against the tendon afterward, you still only twitch briefly, not continuously. That wouldn't make any sense, and your body (specifically, your brain) knows it. So the mighty, mighty CNS regulates your reflexes through this process of modulation.

Okay, **so why is that important to us**? Remember that from one thing, we learn ten thousand things. We can consciously control how often our neural patterns fire, if they fire, to what extent they fire, etc.... **but only through conscious effort**. In other words, our higher brain functions are capable of regulating our patterns (habits) with great precision, but only if we pay close attention to them.

We'll see in a moment that this last detail is where the Devil resides, metaphorically speaking, of course. It requires *conscious effort* to modulate our patterns, and as we'll find out, we have a limit as to how much conscious effort we can expend at one time.

For example, if you stare at your knee, I can whack it all day with my rubber tomahawk and never get a twitch. But, if the ghost of Elvis Presley suddenly appears in the corner of the room, and you, quite understandably, look away from your knee to gawk at The King, I could whack you while you're distracted and I'd get the twitch I was looking for.

Your conscious monitoring of your knee-jerk reflex ended, and so now that there wasn't anything preventing that pattern from firing, when you got whacked… you twitched.

More on this later. For now, all we need to realize is that our neurological patterns can be stopped, started, and controlled almost completely by our higher brain centers, but this requires conscious effort. In other words, **once you aren't expending effort on concentrating, you revert back to what is natural and automatic for you.**

CHAPTER 2:
BACK TO THE SIMPLE REFLEX

So the "simple" reflex isn't really so simple... it's really a surprisingly powerful and complex network. But it's still just simple little neurons, hooked together in various patterns, and all they do is conduct an electrical signal from one end of themselves to the other. The power comes in the pattern itself.

Of course, this explanation is necessarily a bit crude. But hopefully this description will help you more easily understand certain principles of how your body works so that you can use this information for your benefit... namely, getting and staying fit.

I'm going to stress this again and again. **Our bodies (and minds) operate according to certain natural laws**, and I'd rather work with nature than against it, just as I'd rather swim with the current of a river rather than against it... you get further, faster, and you're less tired at the end of it.

So what have we learned so far?

- **our actions, physically, are the result of a pattern of individual neurons linked together.**

- **the more complex the action, the more complex the pattern.**
- **each pattern is activated by a specific input that gets the whole thing started.**
- **our patterns are under our complete control, so long as we can expend conscious effort on modulating them.**

Now, from one thing, we will learn ten thousand things.

We've been talking about physical action being the result of a neural pattern or network. But the exact same mechanism exists for our **thoughts** as well; they are the result of a (very complex, obviously) pattern of neurons firing off electrical signals to each other.

And let's take it a step further. Emotions work through the same mechanism… again, all far more complex than the lowly simple reflex, but the principles are the same!

Impossible, you say. *Why, that would take an enormous number of individual neurons, with a ridiculous number of connections between them.* To which I say, we have twelve **BILLION** neurons, give or take a few, each of which has up to a **HUNDRED THOUSAND** separate dendrite branches (connections), which makes for… heck, I don't even know how many possible combinations. Some math wizard might be able to calculate that number, if we even have a number that big in existence.

Suffice it to say, it's a nearly countless supply of possible patterns and networks. And these connections can change as necessary… but once again, I'm getting ahead of myself. More on that soon.

The point is, *everything we are is essentially a sum of our networks and patterns of neurons.* Our thoughts, our actions, our feelings, and most particularly, our **habits of behavior** are a direct result of masses of individual neurons shooting electrical signals around in various web-like patterns.

POSTURE AS A PATTERN

How about an example? Let's take posture.

When posture correction is done, it usually starts with taking a picture of somebody and then drawing a grid on it to show them what a slouching Neanderthal they really are.

The most common postural distortion is Forward Head Posture, which is an incredibly inventive name for keeping your head too far in front of your body. Ever notice how some people always seem like they're looking down at the ground while they walk, instead of where they're going? It's very common, since most of us are hunched over computers and books and desks all day long.

Now, I won't go into why Forward Head Posture (it's also now called "Text Neck") is so problematic… that's beyond the scope of our discussion here.

The point is, we can see neurological patterning at work here. Once people see that picture of themselves from the side, and it looks like they're jutting their heads out like they're doing the Funky Chicken, they usually exclaim, "That's ME?"

You bet, buckaroo. That's why you need to use a picture instead of just eyeballing it and telling the person about their posture… they probably wouldn't believe it unless they actually saw it.

"Well, I'll just pay attention and straighten myself up."

Hey, good luck with that. I can guarantee it won't work. Here's why.

Sure, you could pay extra careful attention to your posture, and consciously modulate (remember that term?) it so that your head is balanced over your shoulders. That'll last about, oh, ten seconds, before you get distracted, and naturally slouch back down into Grunting Neanderthal posture.

You see, your posture is a result of a **pattern**, a set network of neurological connections that determine where you hold your head. And like any pattern, it's activated by a nerve receptor… in this case, special position receptors that determine position (they're called *proprioceptors*, in case you need a big word later on to impress your friends or win a Scrabble game).

These position receptors tell you where your particular bits are floating in space, and in the case of posture, if those bits (the head, in this case) are too far forward, too far backwards, too far left or right… you get the idea.

Here's the trick. Receptors have a funny little property called **accommodation**, which is what it sounds like. Ever jump into a cold lake? You let out quite a scream at first, didn't you? But after a time, that water didn't feel so cold, did it? Back in Pennsylvania, where I grew up, we used to say the water was cold, "but then it warmed up for me." Right. That big giant lake warmed up, just for little old me.

Wrong. What happened was, the receptors for cold in my skin *accommodated*, or got used to, that level of coldness. Then, it registered cold as being "normal", not "cold", so I didn't experience the temperature of the water as being cold anymore.

Most of your receptors work this way. Stick your hand in a hot bucket of water; it'll feel lukewarm after a short while. Put a dime on the back of your hand; a minute later, you won't notice the pressure it exerts on your skin.

In the case of posture, if you hold your head forward for hours a day, for days and weeks and months, those position receptors will accommodate and tell you that Forward Head Posture is normal. In fact, if you take a slouching forward head patient and straighten them up, a lot of times their eyes get big and they swear they think they're going to go over backwards.

Do you see why? Because to those position receptors, 'forward' is now 'normal', and 'normal' is now 'too far back'.

As I said before, you can pay extra careful attention to your posture to change it consciously, but you're swimming against the current. Your posture's natural state (or pattern) is now "slumped forward", and the second you stop paying attention to it (which, of course, you have to do sooner or later) you will return to that natural state.

Remember when the ghost of Elvis showed up in our examination room, distracting you long enough to let me

whack your knee and get a twitch out of you? Same thing.
This is an important concept that we will deal with over and
over. From one thing, learn ten thousand things.

So to correct that lousy posture, it's necessary to retrain and
reset those receptors, which is done through various means
not important to this book. But there's more.

RULES OF NEUROLOGICAL PATTERNS

That heading sounds really important and complicated,
doesn't it? 'Rules of Neurological Patterns'. But all we're
going to talk about, are the mechanisms of stuff you already
know about and deal with every day. There's nothing to it.
But by understanding how it all works under the hood, you'll
know how to use it to your advantage, and swim with the
current instead of against it. Here we go.

We've just seen the basic structure of a network or pattern of
neurons, and the gist of how those little critters operate. Now
we'll take it up a notch.

Patterns of neurons have certain properties that we need to
understand. They can be:

- **CREATED**
- **DESTROYED**
- **CHANGED/ADAPTED**
- **REINFORCED**

This is critical to understand for our discussion here, because
it forms the basis for how we're going to change our

waistlines for the better and get the right kinds of stares on the beach… for the long term.

Creation of a new network of neurons or neurological attachments is nothing more than learning. Watch a child learn to walk, or throw a ball, or do just about anything. Slowly, over time, they learn which neurons need to fire, which need to not fire, and they form the interconnections between neurons to create a pattern that becomes second nature over time.

It becomes second nature over time, because neural networks are also reinforced by repetitive use.   This happens through two basic mechanisms.

HABIT FORMING

In the first, more and more of your neural interconnections are made, until it's very, very easy for that pattern to fire once the correct input is made. If you have a network of friends, each of whom would invite you to a party, and they make friends, who also make friends, and so on, odds are, you're going to get invited to the same party a whole bunch of times, from separate people (different inputs, essentially).

A simpler, if more crude, way to think of it is like adding strands to a spider web; the more strands you add, the stronger the web becomes.

The other way we reinforce patterns is at the actual connection between neurons… the **synapse**. Go ahead and forget that term; it just means the gap where neuron number one ends and meets neuron number two.

But, there is one property here that's important. The big fat
term is **Long Term Potentiation**... hoo-ah, that's a doosie!...
but all it means is this: the more neuron one makes neuron
two fire, something changes at that synapse, that connecting
gap, that makes it easier for neuron one to make neuron two
fire.

Yep. That's it. That whole big term for that little idea. You
can think of it like an athlete "warming up" before practice;
he's making it easier to use those same skills later.

This is how we form habits, which are nothing more than
neural networks that are extremely highly reinforced. In a
way, you can think of walking, or any other common physical
action, as a habit that we constantly reinforce until we take it
for granted. People who are severely injured and need to
learn to walk again have lost the 'habit' of walking and need
to rebuild and reinforce that neural network.

Conversely, neural networks that aren't used very often begin
to degrade over time. Those branchy connections between
neurons begin to retract and disappear.

Pluck the strands from the spider web, and it starts to weaken,
right? And if neuron one doesn't make neuron two fire, ever,
that Long Term Potentiation thing works in reverse... it's like
corrosion forming on a battery connection, slowing down the
transmission of electricity. Now that synapse, that gap,
doesn't want to let neuron one set off neuron two as easily.

We 'get a little rusty' when we don't use our skills, don't we?
The other day, I had to drive a manual transmission car for
the first time in ten years.

It wasn't pretty. I could still do it; there was enough of a pattern left for me to get by, but there were a few upraised middle fingers lifted my way before it was all over.

Also important, perhaps even most important, is our ability to adapt or change neurological patterns. This is one of the most exciting areas of research… neural *plasticity*, the formation of new nerve cells and their connections to other neurons.

For many years, it was believed that the nervous system remained mostly unchanged in the adult from year to year; that is, the actual circuitry, the neural networks didn't change, just how we used them. Now, evidence suggests our CNS is far more adaptive than we ever gave it credit for. You really can teach an old dog new tricks. You simply have to have the desire to do so.

AUTOPILOT VS. MANUAL

There are some hard-wired patterns that we are born with; many of these are automatic functions beyond our control. In other words, we don't have to learn how to digest food or control our heart rate.

And there are some researchers who believe that some of our behavioral patterns are hard-wired and impossible to change. Some believe that all patterns are adaptable, no matter what.

I personally believe that there is a continuum from hard-wired to completely flexible, with the more innate biological functions sitting on the hard-wired side and the more high-order cognitive and reasoning functions on the flexible side of the equation.

This would also suggest that the more hard-wired your patterns are, the more difficult they will be to change. You can dump addiction-type problems here, since a lot of those use biological reward mechanisms to wreck their particular havoc.

You could also add in things like overeating, which has a biological (evolutionary, really) basis as well... the innate desire to eat like a pig now in case of a starvation situation later. I think we can all agree it would be a heck of a lot harder to completely change our diet (which has a biological connection) than it would be to change our favorite brand of underwear (which, generally speaking, doesn't have a biological connection).

A key reason why adaptation is so important is this: **it is far easier to modify an existing pattern than it is to create an entirely new one**. Think of it this way: if I'm great at throwing a football, it's going to be pretty easy for me to learn how to throw a baseball, since these are similar patterns that probably actually share portions of each other's neural networks.

However, having skill with throwing a football isn't going to help me learn advanced calculus any more quickly than normal; there simply isn't any crossover, no similar portions of neural network to 'borrow' from one activity to the other.

Anyone who wants to create lasting change in their life (like going from soft in the belly to flat in the stomach), must change their behavior at the level of the neural network.

Otherwise, you're making the same mistake as those people hoping they can correct their slumping posture by simply relying on willpower and concentration.

It just doesn't work. **This is why fad diets fail**; once the newness and novelty of the diet fade away and the dieter's willpower and conscious effort fail, they're just going to go right back to the same old habits, the same old patterns, the same old diet as before. It's inevitable. It's natural law.

We'll discuss this and the other concepts in further detail later. The key points to remember are:

- **We are neurological creatures, defined and ruled by our CNS (Central Nervous System), which is our Master Computer.**
- **Our thoughts, emotions, habits, skills, and everything else is the result of a series of neural networks or patterns, each with a specific input and output.**
- **These patterns are infinitely adaptable and can be created, destroyed, reinforced, or changed to meet our needs.**
- **We can control our patterns and networks through conscious effort, but only as long as we can pay close attention to them.**

Chapter 3:

Willpower And Stress

Now that we've seen how neural patterns and networks work, let's see why we have so much trouble changing them into what we want them to be. As I ranted a bit about earlier, a key problem is that we rely far too much on willpower to force us to modulate our behavior, and then kick ourselves when that willpower fails.

But what is willpower, really? If we break it down to its constituent components, what does it look like under the microscope?

Willpower is, essentially, the capacity to do that which is not natural or normal behavior for us. If we're a habitual smoker, when we get the urge to take a drag, we light up a cigarette. But if we're quitting smoking, when we get the urge, we stop the pattern that is natural to us (smoking) and force ourselves to do what is unnatural to us (not smoking).

That's right, folks. All that willpower is, is our ability to consciously modulate our natural patterns of behavior.

That's it. That's all. Nothing mystical or magical or morally superior. For all that we like to celebrate willpower as some sort of majestic superpower, it really just boils down to the utterly common and mundane: conscious modulation, or "focus".

So why is it so hard? After all, the reason why we value willpower so greatly is that so few of us seem to have it... or more accurately, have as much of it as we'd like to.

NO MORE CHANGE, PLEASE... I'M FULL!

There's a psychological/neurological concept called **channel capacity**, which is the idea that our little noggins can process a certain amount of information coming in from several channels at once; that is, several sources at one. Parents think their kids are nuts when they play computer games while watching TV and texting their friends.

We all do it, every day, and in fact, we rely on it for some of our more complex tasks... you know, like driving your car while putting on lipstick and talking on your cell phone and eating your WaWa breakfast bagel all at the same time. Don't lie. I've seen you do it.

Our minds are beyond amazing, beyond incredible, and in the end, perhaps beyond comprehension, at least in their entirety. Every one of us, barring those stricken by serious disease or injury, are capable of processing multiple cognitive inputs from multiple sensory modalities (sight, hearing, touch, etc.), and not only respond to them, but prioritize and then respond to each... or even several at once!

Our lower-level neurology works the same way. You process simple sensory input by the bucketful every second; from the pressure of the seat on your butt to the slight draft blowing across the hairs of your arm to that pesky bug bite on your ankle that won't stop itching to the postural sensors telling you that you're leaning too far back in your chair and are about to fall and bust your head wide open.

Notice, however, a part of the term we're discussing is **capacity**. As in, there's a limit. We're amazing, but come on, cut us a break. We're still only human.

A good example of this comes from people who have sustained injuries in a car crash. It isn't uncommon for whiplash injury victims to suffer any of a number of neurological (and psychological) complaints. Not surprising, since their brains just took a serious jolt.

Some researchers believe that there is a loss of channel capacity in these patients. Let's say pre-accident, John Doe could process cognitive input coming from five sources at once… let's say, his car radio, the actual driving of the car, the song he was singing while the radio plays commercials, his wife talking to him from the passenger seat, and the guy flipping him the bird from the next lane over for not letting him cut in.

After the accident, John's channel capacity cuts down to four channels. Now, in the same example, once that guy in the other lane gives John the one finger salute, John will find he's soon on the receiving end of a cold stare from his wife, since he can't remember a darn thing she's been saying.

Again, this is a complex and in-depth explanation of a phenomenon we are all familiar with. Ever say this: "I've got too much on my mind"? Or, maybe, "I've just got too much on my plate right now"?

No, never, right? What's happening is, your channel capacity has become overloaded. It doesn't have to be from injury or disease. Stressful situations soak up channel capacity like a sponge.

A CHANNEL BY ANY OTHER NAME...

Actually, I don't much like the term channel capacity. I think it implies that we use our neural potential in big chunks, when I believe a continuous pool is more of an accurate metaphor.

After all, with channel theory, a stressful input could only take up one channel, since it's just one thing, leaving you plenty of other channels to access. In my experience, extremely stressful situations overload our capacity **in its entirety**, leaving us incapable of thinking of anything but whatever is causing our stress.

Ever get called into the boss's office, right after you get the word a bunch of people are about to get fired? You're not processing much except anxiety just then, are you?

In any case, the point is this: we have a certain capacity, a limit on how much our neurology can handle at one time. This includes a capacity for conscious modulation, which as we recall, is what willpower actually boils down to.

Can we all see the importance of this implication? We have, by our very nature, by the physical laws that govern our minds and bodies, *an inherent limit to what we call willpower*.

It's built in. You can't avoid it. **So when you overload your system, your system will fail, and you will go back to your natural habits**. It's not weakness. It's natural law.

Remember when we talked about neural patterns and how they can be changed? We change them by reinforcing, through use, the pattern we want to become natural to us.

In order to reinforce a different pattern than we have today, we have to use our cognitive modulation and focus on that change so that we can start reinforcing a new pattern. The bigger the change in behavior, the more of that focus (our "willpower" resource) we will have to expend.

With more and more repetition, that new pattern becomes the norm, the standard, the natural behavior for us. Easy, right? Except…

STRESS

Oh, there it is. The killer. The big Kahuna wrecking-ball that screws up everything. You see, stress… emotional stress… eats up our resources for conscious modulation like pigs at a trough.

Since conscious modulation is merely our ability to focus on changing our natural behavior, **anything that takes up our attention will distract us and steal our focus from changing our behavior.**

Makes sense, right? If I'm working on changing my diet and the room catches on fire, I'm suddenly no longer concerned with how many grams of carbs I've eaten that day. Not burning to death in a fiery inferno has captured my entire attention… as it should! In channel capacity parlance, all the channels are tuned to the same station.

Now, in this example, once the fire is out, or we run out of the building, the stress is over, our capacity is back to normal, and we can happily count our carbs the live-long day. Right? Except real life isn't so cut-and-dried as my over the top metaphor.

In real life, our stresses tend to be chronic. We worry. We worry about what we'll do with our lives, about our jobs, our families, will we succeed, will we fail, and what will come tomorrow. This constant and unrelenting stress has a number of detrimental physical effects which are beyond the scope of this book.

The point is, our stress levels in modern life are soaking up so much of our cognitive resources, that it's not a surprise when people fall off of the wagon with new diets or exercise or what have you. It's a surprise that anyone succeeds, ever!

BIGGER IS NOT BETTER

Remember, the more unnatural a new behavior pattern is (the more we try to change) the more cognitive modulation is required. This is the critical component as to why most weight loss programs fail, and why yours will succeed.

If we use up, say, a third of our focus, our cognitive capacity, on normal day-to-day routine matters, and push ourselves to the limit with the other two-thirds by massively changing our behavior, what happens when a Big Stress Event comes along?

We've already seen the answer to that. The diet fails. We revert back to our old habits, usually in dramatic fashion, and fire down gobs of ice cream or pizza or whatever and spiral down into dejection and despair.

Why we fail so dramatically (rather than just a little) is a topic we'll cover in a little bit. But now you see how we've come to the mechanism of how our best-laid plans for trimming the fat go awry.

In fact, at this point, I hope you can see how any program that relies on massive, immediate change is doomed to fail. It probably seems a little ridiculous now, doesn't it?

Expect a couch potato who's been reinforcing a pattern of fast food and inactivity for forty years to jump up, turn 180 degrees to everything that is natural and ingrained into their life, and maintain that total change indefinitely regardless of what else is going on in their life?

Ridiculous. Insane. Impossible. Oh, it happens, from time to time. On rare occasion, somebody will totally turn their life around and actually stick with it in the long term.

How do they do it? They ignore everything else in their life, usually. They de-prioritize everything not related to diet and exercise, and literally live for just that. It frees up their channel capacity to such an extent that they can fill it all up with nothing but changing their fitness behavior.

Unfortunately, not all of us have this luxury. Not all of us can simply ignore or set aside everything else in life just to get a rock-hard six-pack. We have responsibilities. We have a life! All of existence is not about our body fat, after all.

So what does that mean for our discussion? Well, the answer is fairly simple. If we expect to make a change that sticks… one that we can continuously reinforce over and over, until it becomes the natural pattern of behavior… it can't be too drastic. **If the change is too big, as soon as the stresses of everyday life surge, our focus will naturally fail and we will revert back to our old pattern**.

If we keep the change small, however, the drain on our cognitive capacity is also smaller, and therefore more likely to survive a surge in stress. We will be able to continually reinforce our new behavior until it becomes the new natural pattern, and then we can move on to the next level.

As we'll soon see, this is how we will step our way one bit at a time to where we want to be, without overwhelming ourselves. We do that by breaking down a large goal into smaller, progressive mini-goals. But before we can talk about breaking a goal down, first we have to talk about goals themselves.

Let's summarize the last few chapters before we move on to goal setting.

- **We are the result of adaptive neural patterns which determine our behavior, some of which have been reinforced so many times that they become second nature… reflexive.**
- **To change this behavior requires conscious modulation (we call it "willpower") for which we**

have an inherent limitation or capacity. The more drastic the change, the greater the strain on that capacity.

- Other life events can also take up that focus, and use it up so that we cannot use it for modulating (changing) our behavior any longer. This is where "willpower fails".
- By reducing how much we try to change, we reduce our need for cognitive resources (willpower) so if there is a surge in stress in our lives, we can continue to change our behavior towards our goals.
- After enough reinforcing, these new patterns will become the natural pattern and no longer require willpower to maintain.

CHAPTER 4:

GOAL SETTING: THE BASICS

You can't get someplace until you decide to go there. Similarly, you can't make a change in your life without deciding what that change will be.

What we're talking about here, of course, is **goal setting**. Now that we've discussed the basics of how our neurology works, we can look at the basics of goal setting and apply our new-found knowledge to creating, reaching, and even surpassing those goals.

Goal setting is actually a surprisingly difficult skill, which is a problem, since it's also incredibly important. Improper goal setting is quite possibly the number one killer of weight loss programs out there… and if you think about it, it makes sense; if you head off down the wrong path, it doesn't matter how quickly or efficiently you run. You're just getting to the wrong place that much more quickly!

First off, let's recall that our fitness (or fatness) level at any particular time is a habit, the result of a pattern of behavior. Since the habit is what produces the result, it makes sense to concentrate our efforts on the habit, doesn't it?

Then we get the results we want, sort of as a bonus, and since we keep the habit indefinitely, we keep the results indefinitely as well. Let's take a closer look.

BE-DO-HAVE

A common descriptive device used in self-help is the phrase "Be-Do-Have". I'm not sure where it originated, or who first strung those three words together like that, but like everything else, it's simply a convenient way of expressing an old, old concept.

It works like this: most people focus on results, what they want to "have". They don't care how they get thin, or rich, or whatever. They just want to be there, and that's where they make their mistake.

Instead of focusing on the "have", or the results, **we should instead be focused on the "be", or the process**. From that, we will

BE the person we need to be
      to **DO** the actions we need to take
           to **HAVE** the things we want to have

See what I mean? Let's have an example. By "Being"… let's say, a "healthy person", we'll "Do" the things a healthy person does, like exercise regularly, eat properly, and so forth, and then we'll "Have" the things a healthy person has… let's say, a result like "having super-fantastic awe-inspiring abs".

If all we do is focus on "abs"… the "Have"… then we go on fad diets or take caffeine pills that make our hearts go pitter-pat a little too quickly or whatever, and as soon as we get our "Have" and become thin, we give that crazy nonsense up and go back to our old habits… and therefore, after a little while, our old waistlines. Remember, our physique is the result of our habits, what we do every day.

Natural law, folks. You can't fight it… not for long, at least.

However, if we change our lifestyle, by re-defining who we are… the "Be"… then we will "Have" what we want. Why?

Because when we re-define who we are, we change our patterns of behavior, our habits (that's the "Do"), and once our patterns are changed, then it becomes natural to do what's necessary to get what we want ("Have").

Willpower fails. It has to. We get tired, or depressed, or discouraged, or distracted, or just plain old overwhelmed, and when that happens… yep. You guessed it. We go back to what's natural. What's innate. What's patterned into our neurological make-up.

So forget willpower; or at least, don't rely on it to get you where you need to go. That's swimming upstream.

Better to change the way your patterns are set, and then when you get tired or overwhelmed or depressed, your natural pattern is still to do the proper, goal-oriented thing.

Who's better off? The person whose habit it is, once depressed, to burn through a half-gallon of mint chocolate chip ice cream, or the person whose habit it is, once depressed, to head into the gym and exercise for an hour?

It's really no different, folks… just one habit versus another, one neurological pattern versus another, one output versus another… so you might as well create and reinforce the pattern that's going to help you get that flat stomach.

So when we set our goals, **we focus on the process**, not the result. That way, we keep working toward changing and reinforcing the habits we need to get the results we desire.

We don't set a goal to "lose ten pounds". We set a goal to "cut sugar out of our diet"… and then, when we lose that ten pounds as a result of our new habit, we keep it off… because we keep reinforcing the habit, forever.

AND NOW… IN REVERSE!

Here's something kind of interesting. That little Be-Do-Have idea? It works in reverse, too.

The first time I ever saw this concept expressed, it was with the phrase "Act as If". That'll work as a starting point.

What we're dealing with is basically Have-Do-Be. If we "act as if" we're already the kind of person we aspire to be, then we mimic that kind of person's behavior, which creates a habit (remember, that's the 'Do'), which helps change how we define ourselves (the 'Be').

Here's how that last part works. We often define ourselves by our actions; in other words, if we find ourselves acting responsibly on a consistent basis, we say to ourselves, "Hey, look at me! I must be a responsible person."

Or, if we lay around all day eating corn chips in front of the TV, we look at ourselves and say, "Jeesh, look at me. I'm a couch potato."

Self-perception and self-talk are powerful agents in our minds. If you keep telling yourself you're a loser, guess what? You'll find a way to be a loser. If you keep telling yourself you can quit smoking if you really try, you'll do it. It's almost like a form of autosuggestion, or self-hypnosis, in which we change ourselves through simply willing it so.

Here's an interesting little tidbit. Athletes who simply think about performing their sport… that is, they visualize in great detail going through the motions of whatever their sport is… end up performing at a higher level than those who do not visualize in this way.

Those who actually physically practice do the best, obviously, but even just the simple act of visualizing yourself doing something makes you better at it.

Why? Because you're reinforcing patterns. Your mind is a massive, complex network of patterns, for physical and mental and emotional activities, and when you activate that pattern… even just in your mind… you reinforce it.

And when you reinforce it, you make it stronger, more natural, more a part of you. Don't ignore the power of visualization in reaching your goals… or in sabotaging your efforts.

Of course, words aren't enough. Our minds are sophisticated enough that reality will intrude upon the most earnest auto-hypnotist.

Sooner or later, you have to actually walk the walk. And as you do, you'll find yourself defining your personality differently; as somebody who not only can do the things you want to do, but actually does them.

Here's an example. Let's use that "awesome abs" persona and see if we can't autosuggest that to ourselves. Remember one of the goals we wanted, one of the "Have's" we were shooting for, was "get super-fantastic awe-inspiring abs".

And in Be-Do-Have, to get there, we had to "Be" the healthy person, which then trickled down to have us automatically do the right actions, form the right habits and keep them in order to get what we wanted.

Now, in reverse. We go out and we buy the clothes we intend to fit into. We schedule a vacation in the Caribbean, where we're going to walk on the beach with our nice svelte physique. We do things like ab crunches, and read books and magazines on exercise, and start cutting our previously massive portion sizes at meals.

These are not yet habits. Some of them are related to results, like the clothes and the trip, and some are actions, in which we're simply going through the motions of that 'fantastic abs' persona.

The point is, we're acting "as if" we're already there, already where we need to be, and in doing so, we are *emulating* that ideal we're shooting for. Add some visualizations in, and soon, we're going to start looking at ourselves (on a subconscious level, of course) and defining ourselves as "someone with fantastic abs"… because we're already doing many or all of the things a toned and defined person does!

Hero worship is another form of this device, and is a powerful tool that should not be ignored.   When I was growing up and learning to exercise in a gym, I read Arnold Schwarzenegger's book on bodybuilding.

I would look at the photos of him posing and think, "Someday I'll be built like that." Now, I never got into competitive bodybuilding, so I never went that far with my physical training, but the point is, emulating Arnold's physique and training regimen got me started on building a pattern of daily exercise I maintain to this day.

You don't have to match your hero's accomplishments identically; you only need to use that image to jump start your neural networking, until your own self-talk takes over.

FORMING HABITS IN TWO DIRECTIONS

Remember that we are neurological creatures, collections of neural networks and patterns that determine our habits, our thoughts, our emotions, everything.

I'm going to keep repeating this concept over and over, and why? Because I want to reinforce that concept in your mind as much as possible, and repetition is the way to do that.

We learn by creating a new pattern… or adapting an old one… and then reinforcing that pattern through using it over and over again. Physically, mentally, and emotionally, **what we practice is who we are**. That's "Do" leading to "Be". What we practice also determines our results. That's "Do" leading to "Have".

For Have-Do-Be, we retrain the network by emulating what we want to be and then repeating that behavior over and over until it becomes a habit, a pattern, and by forming that pattern, we then begin to define ourselves through self-perception as the kind of person who has those habits in the first place. Building the new networks essentially builds a new you.

The new you then reinforces those habits with self-talk… "That's the kind of person I am"… and so those habits no longer take any effort to sustain. It's now the natural thing to do, like water flowing downhill, so now you're swimming with the current rather than against it.

Rather than simply trying to create the patterns you need to by working in the Be-Do-Have direction, get your results exponentially more quickly by working in the reverse direction as well. You'll be surprised how quickly you make changes in your life… and changes that last.

THE MAKING OF A GOOD GOAL

Now that we know to work on process goals vs. results goals, let's take a look at what makes a good goal. Solid, proper goal setting insures the following characteristics are present in any goal:

SIMPLE
REALISTIC
DEFINITE

We're going to see that these seemingly separate elements of goal setting blend together somewhat, but we'll keep them separate for ease of discussion.

KEEPING IT SIMPLE, STUPID!

There's a popular saying when it comes to planning: KISS, for Keep It Simple, Stupid. And quite frankly, it's the A-Number One rule for any sort of planning, for obvious reasons... the simpler the plan is, the less there is to go wrong.

We've all heard of Murphy's Law... what can go wrong, will go wrong, and at the worst possible time... and KISS minimizes Murphy's ability to heave monkey wrenches into our best-laid plans.

In the case of goal setting, keeping things simple serves additional functions, as well. First off, it makes your job easier and less stressful (remember what we just said about stress). It's easier to create a simple plan for a simple goal. Seems pretty self-evident, right?

Here's why that's so important. We're pretty fickle creatures, we humans. We tend to take things a little too seriously sometimes, particularly failure (I myself am a terrible culprit of this).

And so, when we embark on something new, especially something experimental (which, by definition, is what changing our lifestyle means) the littlest setback puts us at great risk for simply throwing up our hands and setting fire to the whole experiment. *Forget this junk*, we say. *That doesn't work at all!*

Is it right to do that? Nope. Is it smart? Nope. Is it functional, rational, reasonable, helpful, productive? Nope to all. Do we all do it?

Heck, yes, we do! It's called nature, folks, human nature, and as I keep saying, we can either fight it and swim upstream or work with it and swim with the current. You choose.

For me, I'll pick swimming with the current each time. It's too darn discouraging to do anything else.

So instead of fighting our human nature, which is to give up on forming a new pattern of behavior easily, we'll work with it (more on not beating ourselves up over giving up on new patterns of behavior soon). First off, we'll give ourselves far fewer opportunities for failure, by making a simple goal and a simple plan to get there.

Another reason for simple goals is this… it's more honest. We have built within ourselves a sort of Censorship Bureau, or Editing Department. That's not a bad thing; it keeps you from saying inappropriate little tidbits like "Wow, that's an ugly kid you've got there!" or "So, are you pregnant or just fat?"

But it also tends to edit the way we think about certain things. A conscience is a great tool for keeping you out of trouble, but it can also serve to stifle your true emotions, and your true ambitions.

Maybe you would really like to get in better shape for the reason most of us do: to look better naked. But your internal sensor won't let you admit that; no, no, you're getting in better shape to, uh, lower your cholesterol level, or maybe, improve your resting heart rate… yeah! That's it! A lower resting heart rate!

Of course that's nonsense. We know that's not why you're doing what you're doing. And the problem you run into, if you're not honest with what you really want and why you really want it, is that you start misdirecting your energies toward the pretty lie rather than the stark truth... which, of course, then means you're not going after what you REALLY want to go after... only what you're willing to *admit* to wanting to go after.

The simpler you keep your goals, the less likely you are to try to censor or edit yourself or otherwise make your goals more Politically Correct from a psychological point of view.

Simplicity is hard to argue with and hard to lie to; so keep your goals simple, and they will be more likely to truly reflect what you want, and not just reflect what you're willing to admit you want.

Simple goals also tend to be a bit more realistic, which is what we'll discuss next.

KEEPIN' IT REAL

This is, without a doubt, the biggest, nastiest, hairiest pitfall of them all when it comes to goal setting. More people fail in their endeavors, their relationships, their careers, and their lives because of this above all other mistakes in choosing goals.

Yes, we should all reach for the stars, and all that lovely poetic hoo-ha. But to reach the stars, you have to build a hell of a ladder first, or you're going to fall flat on your face, which happens all too often when someone sets a lofty and unrealistic goal.

It's simple. Failure is disheartening. As we'll see in a moment, failing to reach a goal has a nasty habit of spiraling down into despair, frustration, and plain old giving up.

So let's avoid all that as much as we can, and start by setting goals we might actually be able to achieve in our lifetime. Sure, we'd all like to have the perfect body, but seriously… are you willing to take the time? The energy? The commitment?

Don't be fooled by the pictures of fitness gods and goddesses you see on the covers of magazines. Most people are never going to get into that kind of shape… and that's okay. Know why? Because *those people look good for a living*. It's their job to look perfect, and believe me, they work at it.

I've known quite a few bodybuilders and fitness models. These people are usually in the gym every day, sometimes for hours at a time. They are obsessive about their diets, to the point where it consumes much of their daily life.

How much of that are you up for? The amount of effort and dedication you're willing to put into this is going to determine your results… so if you're not willing to do five days a week of cardio training, resistance training, and abs training, and six days a week of eating a whole foods diet with one Cheat Day… you're not going to get a body like someone who WILL do those things. Which is fine, by the way… just keep your expectations in line with what you're willing to do (and sacrifice) in order to meet those expectations.

The point is this. You have inherent limitations in your life. You only have so much time. You only have so much energy.

You only have so much focus… remember cognitive capacity? So keep those in mind when setting your goals. Keep your feet on the ground.

That doesn't mean give up. That just means, if you can't do the lifestyle I just described, maybe set a goal that's a little more realistic. You can still lose weight, get trim, and look good with a lesser program than what I just described… you just won't be ready for the cover of a magazine. And if you're okay with that, I'm okay with that. I just want you to get a realistic idea of what's involved, so you can set your goals accordingly and not be misled.

There is another complicating factor to consider, as well. Genetics.

I hesitate to mention this, because unfortunately, too many people use genetics as a crutch or get out of jail free card, an excuse to give up and stay fat and out of shape. "Oh, I was born fat. I'll always be fat."

Nothing could be further from the truth. Everyone… EVERYONE… can improve their fitness level, no matter what their genetics are.

However… it is true that some people will have a harder time than others. Some people are naturally lean, some are naturally heavy. We each vary in our bony framework, as well. Some women practically starve themselves to death, worried about the size of their hips, when they are already as lean as lean can be. Not everyone has a tiny pelvis like a runway model. You can't change your bony framework.

Again, avoid the temptation to use this as an excuse to throw in the towel. If you aren't genetically blessed, you can still make a big difference in your body shape with proper diet and exercise… just temper your expectations with the knowledge that you might not get results as quickly and easily as the next person. Don't give up… just be realistic.

BE DEFINITIVE

The last thing I want to discuss about goal setting is the importance of setting *definite* goals. Not only are hazy goals clumsy to work with, they're deadly to our momentum of success. Here's why.

First off, a hazy goal is difficult to break down into sub-goals. They're also difficult to assess as far as what's reasonable, and what's not. Let's pick a hazy goal and see what we're talking about here.

"I want to be rich."

Okay. Great. Nothing wrong with that goal… at least, not on the surface. Let's take a closer look, though, and see that our apparently simple and distinct goal is really neither.

First off, what's rich? A million dollars? Ten million dollars? A billion jillion dollars? And do we even define rich in terms of a big chunk of money, or in the income that an investment portfolio of that size would produce?

Why do we want to be rich? Is it to snub our noses at the neighbors? It's maybe best not to dedicate one's efforts to such a poorly motivated goal. Is it because we want financial security? A big house? A collection of artwork that would

turn a museum green with envy? And do we need to actually
be rich to have those things?

How about sub-goals, which we'll discuss in a moment? If we
have no idea what our actual destination is, how can we
possibly plan stepping stones in order to get there?

We can start seeing several pitfalls in our hazy goal of "I want
to be rich". Most important, though, is this problem: how do
you know when you've gotten there? When can you declare
victory, pat yourself on the back and say, "Yep! I'm rich!
Success at last!"

It doesn't matter if we simply make progress; we have to be
able to **mark** our progress, keep score, and actually validate
our efforts in a definitive and obvious way. Otherwise, we
don't emotionally feel like we're getting anywhere.

We need that unambiguous, clear, undeniable affirmation that
we're going in the right direction. Only then do we
congratulate ourselves on a job well done and push onwards
and upwards.

So, we know we need to draw a finish line, with no doubt as
to where that finish line lies. In the case of our "get rich" goal,
perhaps once we examine our reasons behind our goal, we
realize that what we really need is to "create an investment
portfolio that generates five thousand dollars a month in
passive income".

We can see that this is a much more definite, clear goal than
simply "get rich". Yet, it's still simple and straightforward
enough that we can begin to subgoal it with ease.

Of course, there's nothing to say that, once we reach our finish line, we can't pick another finish line and run for that one next… once we catch our breath, of course.

In the above example, after we reach our five-grand-a-month goal, a nice little vacation would definitely be in order, and then perhaps a new goal of eight or ten thousand a month is certainly reasonable at that point.

This example is not fitness-related, obviously, but you can easily see how this principle can be used in determining six-pack-abs related goals. It's terribly important, especially when it comes to motivation, as we'll see in the next chapters.

Realistic, simple, definite goals, broken down into stepping stones we can rapidly achieve. Now you know why it works; now you can make it work for you.

So what have we learned in this chapter?

- **Focus on process goals, not results goals. By focusing on the process, we not only get the results, we keep them, because we don't go back to our old habits once we reach that magic number of pounds or inches or whatever.**
- **By keeping our goals simple, realistic, and easily defined, we make achieving our goals much easier, and make the process of breaking down those goals easier as well.**

Chapter 5:

Stepping Stones To Success

Now that we've talked a little about goal setting, let's recall that the more change we make in our lives, the more willpower… which is just our ability to focus on and cognitively modulate our natural pattern of behavior… we will need. Also recall that since stress eats up that same resource, if we want a new pattern of behavior to stick, we need to minimize that change, minimize the amount of willpower involved, in order to maximize the odds that we will stick with our new habits.

Changing your lifestyle can be a daunting task. It's too much to take on at one shot… remember the old joke I mentioned earlier about "How do you eat an elephant?" One bite at a time.

Any more than that, and you'll choke… become frustrated and give up. So when you go to make big lifestyle changes in order to improve your fitness, you're going to need to break any big, lofty goals down into much more palatable, bite-sized pieces.

These pieces are called sub-goals or stepping stones, and they're what they sound like. We take a great big goal and break it down into smaller, easier to achieve goals.

Want to lose fifty pounds? Better start with ten, and then
another, and then another, until you finally hit your larger
goal of fifty. See what I mean? Of course, we're ignoring my
advice that we shoot for process goals rather than results
goals, but you get the idea.

Breaking up a large goal into smaller sub-goals makes
achieving results occur more quickly. It also makes things a
lot easier to manage, as well. Some goals have multiple,
complex components to achieve.

Becoming a millionaire is a big goal, not just numerically, but
in the sense that it will (in most cases) require learning a
number of skills in order to reach it. Breaking something like
that down into sub-goals organizes your efforts and
streamlines them.

Remember, the simpler things are, the easier they are. Life is
tough enough. Make it as easy for you as you can.

This isn't a difficult concept to grasp, but it is vital to your
success with any weight loss or fitness endeavor. Rome
wasn't built in a day, and a chubby couch potato doesn't turn
into an Adonis overnight. If you've got a long way to go,
you're going to have to make small changes over time if you
expect them to last.

In fact, at this point in our discussion, it's probably become
evident that this is where most diet and exercise programs
fail… they neglect to allow for small enough change over a
long enough time to give your neurology a chance to adapt,
change, and make the new behavior the natural response.

This is how your program will succeed where others have failed. Now that you know that undertaking too much change too quickly overwhelms the nervous system… and why that happens… you can avoid that pitfall and make your new fitness program stick around for the long term.

The basics of how to do this are fairly self-evident. If you have a large, significant goal, you simply split it up into smaller bits. Simple, right? But so few of us do it! We all dive right in to "I want to be perfect" and never acknowledge the separate steps that's going to require.

So the first trick with stepping stones is to actually use them! It may seem like a silly intellectual exercise, but believe me, it's not. There's countless reasons to break large, unwieldy goals down, as we'll see through the next chapters. So first, actually use these sub-goals.

The next trick with stepping stones is to make sure that they lead back to where you are today… the starting point. Always remember that **you can't start anywhere but where you are right now**, so if you're a little embarrassed about your current state of fitness, you're going to have to get over that when you assess where you are today. Otherwise, you won't be able to figure out how to get where you want to go.

We're going to re-visit this when we measure ourselves in Section 3 of this book. Again, the reason for measurement isn't to embarrass you or make you feel bad about yourself. It's a necessary first step.

If I want to make myself a millionaire, I need to know how much I have in the bank account today in order to know what I'm going to have to do to get to one million dollars.

Similarly, it's important that we assess ourselves today so that we can draw a road map to where we want to be fitness-wise. This may sound simple, but as I just mentioned, some people are a little embarrassed to admit to the actual real size of their waistline.

If we say, "I want to have a 32 inch waist", it makes a big difference in the amount of lifestyle change if we are currently at a 42 inch waist versus a 34 inch waist. See what I mean?

Think of those mental stepping stones, as stepping stones across a river. And just like in a river, you have to make sure your smaller goals lead from where you are on this side of the river, to where you want to go on the other side, without any gaps too big to jump.

HOW SIMPLE IS SIMPLE?

Remember when we said our goals have to be simple? How simple are they, really? You might be surprised. Let's say that I have a goal we'll call "**HEALTHY PERSON**". But…

"**BETTER DIET**" might be just one part of that goal…

… and "**LESS JUNK FOOD**" might be just one part of "**BETTER DIET**"…

…and "**LESS PIZZA FOR LUNCH**" might be just a part of "**LESS JUNK FOOD**"!

Those who know me know that I used to have a serious problem with an addiction to a local pizza shop. Changing

that pattern in and of itself was a daunting, daunting task…
and it's still not eradicated (remember our talk on Cheat
Days?)!

Seriously, though, looking at how an apparently simple goal
breaks down into other goals, each of which breaks down into
at least one more goal, we can see how suddenly, we're trying
to tackle what turns out to be 157 goals at once when we
thought it would be only one.

In this case, just that one goal would exhaust our channel
capacity for change… and perhaps even overwhelm it. And,
of course, human nature dictates that we would never
recognize this, but simply get frustrated and give up.

Keeping your goals simple and breaking them down into
smaller goals will help you to avoid this form of channel
capacity burnout and give you a realistic idea of how much
you're actually taking on at once. Another side benefit of this
is that you'll be more easily able to prioritize what steps you
need to be taking at any particular time in order to follow
your prescribed path.

The process of sub-goalling itself allows us to not only
examine our overall, lofty goals and decide not only if we're
taking on too much at once, but also which parts of our
stepping stones are most important to take on first and second
and third.

Be careful to examine your goals to insure that they don't
actually break down into many simpler ones… and don't try
to change too many areas of your life at once. You'll only set
yourself up for disaster.

RECYLING AN OLD PATTERN

Recall earlier in our discussion of neurological patterns that we discussed a term called *plasticity*. If you remember, that's just a really grandiose term for learning… but a particular neurological component of learning.

If we think of our neural networks as spider webs creating a distinctive pattern between set points, we get a decent analogy for the multiple connections between each of our twelve billion neurons. Each neuron can be thought of as a dot in the page, and each connection as a line from one dot to another. Now add another and another and another, and you get your spiderweb, your distinct pattern.

Let's say you need to refine your pattern. It's close to what you want, but not quite exactly there. Rather than start over, you erase a line here, add one there… maybe even change up some of the dots. This is plasticity… changing the actual, physical makeup of your neural network in order to refine your patterning.

It isn't hard to imagine the changes taking place in a stumbling child, desperate to learn to walk unaided (no doubt if only to knock over a potted plant while Mom's not looking). At first, the spiderweb-like pattern is barely there; only a few lines connecting even fewer dots. Then more lines are added, and more, as the child finally stands up and takes that first step.

BAM! They fall down. Need a little refinement, there. So we erase a few of those lines, try some new ones… form some new connections.

BAM! Okay, that wasn't it either. Now a few other lines are added, a few more removed, and this time, the child wobbles a bit after that step, but doesn't fall. And so the process continues, as that neural network gets some connections added, and others weeded out, until we have the network for walking perfected.

How does this apply to us? Often, it's easier to adapt an existing pattern than to create a new one, and sometimes, there's no choice BUT to shift an existing pattern.

If we can simply modify an existing pattern of behavior, there's less effort… always a good thing… required to get to our goals. **Remember, quick and easy goals, achieved with as little frustration as possible, arranged in stepping stones from where we are today to where we want to be, is the cornerstone philosophy of true, long term fitness success.**

An old expression is "play to your strengths". One way you can do this is to start any new change in your life by simply nudging current behavior in a better direction. Here's an example.

Let's say I want to eat a healthy diet, but I currently eat lunch every day at a pizza shop (which, of course, is not true, and by that I mean, it used to be). If I tried to just scrap my everyday habit and eat nothing but sprouts and carrots, I'd freak out within a week or two and go right back to my good old, solidly reinforced pattern of eating pizza.

Instead, I could take an easy first step, like not drinking soda when I go to the pizza shop. I'll just drink water instead. Not a big change, right? Not going to impress anyone with that. But it IS a change, and a change in the right direction. Once that's a habit, maybe I'll pick one day a week NOT to go to the pizza shop. Four days a week instead of five. And I'll keep reinforcing that habit until it's second nature.

It's not sexy. It's not dramatic. It's not going to get you quickie results like those ridiculous books and magazines that promise LOSE TEN POUNDS IN FOUR HOURS!

What it *will* do, is **work**. Permanently. And you're far more likely to get where you want to go, because you'll hardly notice getting there. It won't be as frustrating, or uncomfortable, or difficult. Stepping stones.

Have you ever gotten sore from a new exercise program, or ever gotten frustrated learning complex math or a new language or just about anything? It's frustrating to learn new things. It's frustrating to change our habits, to re-arrange our neural networks.

It shouldn't be that way, but it is. So don't sabotage yourself by relying on just 'toughing through it' or 'sucking it up' or any of those other concepts that rely on willpower.

Willpower fails. It takes up too much energy, requires too much of our attention, and eventually, it must fail, and we'll just go right back to our old, reinforced patterns. It's natural law.

Too big of steps is one thing. The same problem applies to taking steps too quickly. Our capacity for change doesn't just

go for how big of a single change we can make at a go... we
also have a certain capacity for how much overall change we
can make at once.

THE TIME ELEMENT

When we set goals, sometimes we have a tendency to
overestimate just how quickly we can accomplish something.
Not just how much we can do, but how quickly we can do it.
They're similar concepts with similar consequences, and you
have to watch out for both in your own goal setting.

So often, when we decide we want to make a change in our
lives, we want to make *massive* change, right now, now, now.
It's critical to understand that change, like healing, takes time,
and that we have to learn to use time to our advantage rather
than trying to force ourselves to swallow too much too fast.

Changing our neural networks takes time. It takes time to
grow those new dendrites (remember, the branchy
connections between the neurons).

And at first, those connections will be few and far between...
weak isn't the word. It's barely perceptible. It takes a lot of
time to constantly reinforce that neural network, with more
and more and more connections creating that stronger
'spiderweb' which we call a habit.

This means, of course, that we'll fail at creating our new
habits. Of course we will. We'll sneak cigarettes or pints of
ice cream or skip days at the gym. It's inevitable. It's natural
law... our new pattern just isn't strong enough yet, and the
old pattern hasn't faded enough.

But it's vital that we don't fall into the old trap of berating ourselves, beating ourselves down for 'failing' to live up to yet another unrealistic expectation… of instant change. How could you possibly change overnight? It's a biological impossibility.

It's important to understand this, because now that you know why you stumble and slip when you're making changes in your life, you can stop kicking yourself and making the situation worse.

We all know how that goes. We try to start a new diet, and two weeks into it, we break down and snitch a bag of chips. Oh, man, then the self-hate begins. What a failure we are. What a loser. Why even try.

I call this the **Why Bother** mindset (creative, hunh?) and we'll talk about it further in a moment in the chapter on motivation. It actually has a reason for existence… to keep us from wasting valuable energy… and you need to understand that it's a natural mechanism. A mechanism to be avoided, of course, but it's not your fault it's there.

Blame our species' evolving in a harsh, starvation-prone world. But don't blame yourself. Because once you blame yourself, you hit the Why Bother input button… and when the Why Bother pattern kicks in, you give up.

Your old habits, your existing patterns and networks that you've been reinforcing all of your life, will die hard. No kidding. But now you know that this is NATURAL; it's not your fault for being a horrible, horrible person who is weak-willed and blah, blah, blah.

That's nonsense. You can't possibly expect a new, barely-formed neural pattern with all of two or three connections to compete evenly with an established pattern of perhaps thousands of connections. The very notion violates natural law, and as I've said before many times, it's best to work with natural law rather than against it.

Beating yourself up because your new pattern isn't set in stone yet? That's swimming upstream.

Rather, when you slip, simply recognize the situation for what it is… an old pattern is kicking in, and a new one needs to be reinforced. That's it. That's all. No big drama. No blame.

Just work with the mechanism. Old networks take time to decay, and new networks take time to build up and reinforce. So let them! Have a little faith in yourself and in your biology.

The new pattern WILL form. The old pattern WILL fade. Not over night, but it will happen. It must happen… it doesn't have a choice. It's natural law.

IF IT'S STUPID, AND IT WORKS, IT ISN'T STUPID

A helpful tool in goal-setting, and setting up sub-goals, is actually writing them down. Yes, I know, it seems a little goofy and corny and downright stupid when you're doing it. I feel a little silly writing down my goals sometimes, especially the small ones.

But then I remember one of my favorite sayings, which is the heading for this section. If it's stupid, and it works, it isn't stupid.

And it really does work… if you actually do it. Of course, it isn't enough to just scrawl your goals out onto the back of an old newspaper that you then throw in the direction of the nearest trash can.

When you write down your goals, you have a perfect opportunity to begin breaking them down into smaller, more accessible stepping stones. Plus, you can make them more clearly defined, and all of the other important components of goal setting which we've already discussed.

The point is, writing your goals down will aid you tremendously in your goal setting efforts, which will, in turn, help your motivation. I'm going to talk more about this in the next chapter, and don't try to stop me.

Are you starting to see why I stress the importance of patterns and networks? Do you see how so many pieces connect together over and over again until they become almost indistinguishable?

It's no accident that I keep repeating certain concepts over and over again, or show you how one part is related to another is related to another (or how I keep having to promise to get to certain concepts later, so I don't get lost on a tangent, as I have a habit of doing!).

It's all a network, each part of the web interconnected with and dependent on each other, and also supportive of each other. The more you can adopt one part of the pattern, the more easily you'll be able to adopt the rest, until it all seems so easy, you'll wonder how it was ever any other way. It really is like pulling yourself up by your bootstraps!

To summarize:

- **Set simple, realistic, definite goals that focus on the process rather than the end result. Feel free to monitor your results, but keep your focus on the process.**
- **Break down those goals into smaller stepping stones that lead backward from where you want to be (the big goal) to where you are today.**
- **Give these small steps time to become a natural part of you; i.e., become reinforced until they feel natural, before you move on to the next one. It will take time; let it.**

CHAPTER 6:

MOTIVATION

Ah, here we are at motivation.   I bet some of you were wondering when we'd get around to that.

Ever notice how some people seem to be more motivated? You look at people who have achieved great things in their lives, and you think to yourself, that guy must have 30 hours a day, or maybe eight days a week. How can they get so much more done than I do?

There's a lot of answers to that question, but the most important is motivation. And it isn't that these successful people are more naturally motivated than the rest of us; remember, their bodies, their neurology is subject to the same natural laws as the rest of ours. But they've got more of something the rest of us lack.

Results.

SUCCESS CREATES MOTIVATION

If you put a quarter into a slot machine, and it hit the jackpot, and you did it again, and it hit again, and so on and so forth, after three or four quarters, would you just shrug your shoulders, say "eh, forget it", and walk away?

No way you would! You'd dig out every quarter you had, then pester your neighbor for more after you'd run out, and after that, you'd run around like a nut, looking for more and more quarters, filled with an excitement and an energy that was almost euphoric.

You've seen results, and that has motivated you to take action; because, unlike so many things we do during the day that never seem to make a dent in our lives, NOW you've stumbled across something that actually PAYS OFF.

The reverse is true. How many of us have started on a new path in our lives… let's say, a new exercise program so we'll lose weight and get super sexy… only to give up a week or two later because it isn't doing squat for us? We hate to spin our wheels. Energy spent + no return on investment = one very unhappy camper.

Remember when I mentioned the "Why Bother" pattern? This is what we're talking about. There's a biological reason for it.

For the vast majority of our species' existence, starvation was a way of life. There weren't any supermarkets or refrigerators or preservatives or heck, even Ziploc baggies back in the good old Stone Age when the human body was being shaped by evolution into the form it is today. And evolution created many solutions to the crisis of there never seeming to be enough to eat.

The human body is a conservation specialist; if you don't need it, you don't keep it. Why do you think muscles atrophy… weaken and shrink up… when we don't use them?

Because muscle tissue burns energy just by being there (more on this later in the chapter on exercise), and if you're burning up valuable calories just to have killer biceps, you're going to end up dead, dead, dead in a starvation-prone environment. Survival is the name of the game, so if you don't need those eighteen-inch pythons to keep yourself alive from one day to the next, guess what?

They're going to disappear. And when there's not enough to eat, you should be glad those biceps DID disappear, or they would burn up the calories you require to do all kinds of frivolous things like, say, breathe, or keep your heart beating.

This concept in biology is called "use it or lose it", and now you know why it's there... to keep us alive in a time of famine, which used to be practically all of the time.

Nowadays, we're lucky enough that most of us in the civilized world don't have to worry about famine (exactly the opposite, really) but the natural, biological makeup of our bodies... the genetic base created over all those millions of years of evolution... *hasn't changed a bit.*

You've read this before. From one thing, learn ten thousand things.

If our bodies resist expending energy to maintain useless tissue (like muscles that aren't being used), you can bet our minds aren't going to waste any time burning energy on activities that don't net results. It's not safe, from an evolutionary perspective, to waste our time like that, and remember that our bodies still operate like we're living in the Stone Age.

So people who try something out and don't see results feel like they're just spinning their wheels and they give up. It doesn't matter if it was the right thing to do; it doesn't matter if they actually really were doing everything they should've been doing, and simply needed to stick with it just a little longer. If we don't see results quickly, we tend to give up.

You can spiral down, or spiral up. It's mostly a matter of knowing how to do it. And so goal setting becomes a factor in motivation, and vice versa.

DESPITE SOME PEOPLE'S OPINIONS, WE'RE SMARTER THAN DONKEYS

Goals are not set in stone. I can't stand reading fitness gurus who demand that you beat yourself senseless if you fail to reach your goals. "Use the carrot and the stick", they'll say, which, by the way, is sort of a mixed metaphor.

We all know about the image of getting a stubborn donkey to move forward, by dangling a carrot from a string tied to a stick so that the dumb old donkey constantly walks forward, never reaching the carrot dangling in front of him.

This metaphor is counterproductive for us on many levels, particularly in the hands of clumsy fitness gurus. First off, we're not dumb asses, no matter what the people stuck behind me in traffic might say.

One of the key rules of intervention psychology is that intervention works best when the subject has no idea that an intervention is going on. In other words, **when we know we're being manipulated, we resist... even if that manipulation is for our benefit**.

Don't believe me? Go out and tell somebody to quit smoking… I mean in great detail. They'll nod along and accommodate you until they get finally get irritated and light up and blow a drag right in your face to make you go away.

Do you really think they don't know that smoking is bad for them? Of course they do. But if you slap them in the face with change, they'll fight you. It's just what we do.

So this notion that we can artificially dangle rewards in front of our face, never really getting them, is hogwash. That'll last about ten seconds before us clever humans simply cut the stick and grab the carrot, sitting immovable in the road immediately thereafter.

You have to give yourself rewards, plenty and often, and the best reward is the satisfaction of success. It's yet another reason why **we need to set small, easily attainable goals, arranged in rapid succession in the direction of our larger, overall goals**. We thrive on rewards, so for God's sake, give yourself some!

The other problem with that 'carrot and stick' saying is when a misguided guru somehow forgets that the purpose of the stick in this image is to extend the carrot out of reach, not to beat the crap out of the donkey. According to these folks, 'carrot and stick' means 'rewards and punishments'. Big mistake, boys and girls.

Punishment, as a rule, is a poor motivator. Which is strange, because so much of what we do in order to effect change in behavior, either in ourselves or in others, is based on punishment. Kids are acting up? Spank 'em! Employees at work aren't reaching their quotas? Fire or reprimand them! Your husband isn't taking the trash out? Hit him in the head with an iron skillet!

Reinforcing this misguided notion of using punishment as an effective tool is misunderstanding the lessons of texts like The Art Of War or other military-type texts as they apply to business or private life.

I know, I know, I keep repeating "From one thing, learn ten thousand things", but understand, sometimes the Devil really is in the details, and metaphors can be strained to the breaking point. Here's what I mean.

WE AREN'T IN THE ARMY, NOW

In the military, punishment is slightly more effective as a tool than in the private sector, for this simple reason... power is absolute in the military. There is a higher authority, who cannot be escaped, imposing their will on you, and you have no choice but to submit or suffer.

If you try to escape the situation, you'll be shot as a deserter. See what I mean? Power is an absolute thing in the military. Obey or die, and there's no way out.

This really doesn't exist in the private sector. Even in the case of a job, in which you face the risk of being fired, you still have a way out.

Nobody is going to take constant, severe abuse forever, no matter how good the paycheck... after all, there's always other jobs, other careers, or even just plain old giving up and going on welfare, which may not be seen as a 'solution' to most of us, but for someone desperate to end punishment, even counterproductive behavior starts to look good.

Do you see why we can't apply military thinking on punishment to our lives, at least, not as directly as those 'carrot and stick' gurus propose? Who on Earth, aside from a raving masochist, is going to constantly beat themselves up... voluntarily, mind you... over and over, consistently, even when tired, depressed, burned out, stressed from the occasional disaster that plagues our daily lives, etc., etc.?

Nobody, that's who. Oh, I guess you could recruit somebody to beat you when you're too tired to beat yourself, but hey... WHY WOULD YOU WANT TO?

What kind of miserable life would that be, to constantly get beaten down for failure, failure which is inevitable from time to time, since we're human and therefore fallible?

And don't forget that when we punish ourselves for defeat, we're very forcefully activating our Why Bother pattern. Remember that?

Remember how once it starts, it tends to spiral downward, until it's out of control and we're stuck in the rut of depression? Except now, we have even MORE reason to never bother to try anything... because if and when we do slip and fall, not only do we call ourselves a loser, we have to endure punishment on top of that!

Fantastic idea, isn't it? While you're at it, load up the closest handgun, and shoot yourself in the foot. BOTH feet. Several times.

Punishment is used so often **because it's easy**. It doesn't take much creativity to smack somebody across the back of the head. It does require creativity, however, to provide a reward system that will inspire someone (including ourselves) toward proper action.

Like I said, though, punishment really doesn't work. Not in the long term. You see, we're NOT dumb old donkeys, plodding along completely oblivious to our surroundings.

We're intelligent creatures, self-aware and more clever than we give ourselves credit for. We know we don't like pain, so we do what we can to avoid it… which forms the basis for the entire notion of punishment. Hey, if I tell you I'm going to hit you in the head with a brick if you don't do your homework, you'd have to be nuts not to comply, right?

The irony is, the basis of punishment is the root of its failure. Of course I want to avoid pain. But the punisher assumes that the only way to avoid pain, is obedience. Wrong.

I can avoid the situation entirely… by quitting my job, running away from home, or giving up in any number of ways. Or I can create the illusion of obedience, simply to avoid a beating.

We're creative individuals, not animals, and while animals might respond somewhat to a punishment system of reinforcement, we won't (Actually, those of you with pets know animals are often clever enough to end-run our best disciplinary attempts as well. How many of you have dogs that have somehow figured out how to open or unlatch doors you swore were secure when you left home?). There's a million ways to end-run punishment, and that's not the only way it fails as a mechanism for change.

Punishment is a temporary stimulus. It has to be. An authority figure cannot constantly be present; it's simply impossible. And we all know, that once the cat's away, the mice will play.

Remove that overbearing, authoritative presence, and watch that 'change' you thought you'd created go straight out the window and the old, reinforced, natural pattern re-emerge.

Going back to the example of the military, even in a situation where punishment can be made more effective, wise commanders realize that punishment is very limited in usefulness. After all, even with the harsh spectre of military punishment hanging over their heads, some soldiers still disobey.

STAY POSITIVE

Far more effective is *positive* reinforcement, a reward system. Take, for example, the idea of esprit de corps, or pride in one's unit. Do you think it's just hot air for the Army to bestow 'elite' status on a select group of high achievers… like Airborne troops, or Special Forces, or Rangers, or whatever other unit you like? It may seem silly to some people to jump out of a perfectly good airplane multiple times just to get a patch on your arm, but for those soldiers who choose to go that route… or any other elite unit… it's more than just that patch.

There is a deep sense of pride attached to being recognized as above average. That, my friends, is a very powerful reward, powerful enough to reinforce discipline until it will stand up under the stress of combat… and can you imagine a tougher stress test?

The threat of punishment won't motivate people that powerfully. A reward system, in this case a sense of pride and belonging and brotherhood, will beat punishment any day of the week.

Mostly I've been talking about one person punishing another, but the same principles hold true when we attempt to punish ourselves. It fails, miserably. It has to.

Either we say "The heck with this!" and stop trying to change at all, or we beat ourselves up so badly we throw ourselves into a depression through a lovely ride down Why Bother lane.

STICK TO REWARDS

So forget any nitwit who tells you it's necessary to beat yourself up in order to change your life. Anybody who says that has only a crude understanding of how rewards and punishments work in human beings.

Animals can be trained this way… B.F. Skinner, the father of modern behavioralism (the branch of psychology concerned with rewards and punishment) did some amazing things with this technique. I can recall reading about an experiment in which pigeons were trained to guide missiles, even to the point of out-performing humans.

But they were *pigeons*. They operate on a far cruder level than we do, so okay, in that situation a simple reward and punishment structure may be effective. Children, at very, very young ages may respond briefly to this sort of learning as well, but it doesn't take them long to mature into sufficient complexity to realize when they're being manipulated... and they don't like it any more than we do.

We are far more complex neurologically than a pigeon or an infant, thank goodness. A system of punishment, however well-meaning, is doomed to fail, because we'll outsmart it... even if 'outsmarting' it is counterproductive to the rest of our lives.

It's just the way we're built. Fight Nature at your own peril.

Toss punishment out of the window, and stick to rewards. It works far more effectively, and guess what? It's much more pleasant and fun to work with.

True, it requires a bit more creativity and subtlety, but if you want lasting results that won't disappear as soon as the first bout of stress appears in your life, learn how to motivate yourself with rewards, and you'll succeed.

WE WORK IN CLAY, NOT IN STONE

Another important point related to punishment is that our goals, while firm, should not be set in stone. Remember, nobody really knows exactly how much change a person can handle at any time. So it's quite possible... inevitable, really... that you will either overshoot or undershoot your mark when you set goals.

Undershooting really isn't a problem. Simply explode through that goal and go on to the next level, flush with new confidence and power at the feeling of succeeding more quickly than you anticipated.

Over-reaching, though, creates an obvious pitfall, and another reason to avoid a punishment system of reinforcement. If we can't possibly reach our goals, and yet we're compelled to kick our own butts if we don't reach them... well, can you say Why Bother?

It doesn't take a genius to figure out the problem there. But again, anyone who advocates this sort of hard-line, do-or-die, burn your bridges behind you so there's no turning back sort of mentality in trying to motivate yourself, has completely missed the boat.

That sort of nonsense may sound good on the surface... you know, give the impression of being 'hard-core' or 'take no prisoners' or that sort of thing... but it's swimming upstream.

We all are impressed by a strong work ethic, and I think that's the illusory appeal of these die-hard types of programs. We have to suffer for what we want, right?

Well, certainly any endeavor worth undertaking will involve effort, and we should be willing to work to make it all come together. However, simply suffering for the sake of suffering is sheer madness.

There's always enough work to do. There's always going to be plenty of difficulty in getting what you want, all by itself, with no extra help from you.

I've said it before; life is tough enough. Don't make things harder on yourself. Work smarter, not harder, and you'll get where you want to go faster, more efficiently, and you'll be happier while you do it!

And isn't that what really counts, folks? What's the point of looking fantastic if you make yourself constantly, utterly miserable while you do it? Swim with the current, learn to use the natural laws of your body and neurology to your benefit, and get great abs while actually enjoying your life!

OH, WAIT… NOW I ACTUALLY HAVE TO DO IT?

Yes, now that we know what to do and how to do it, we have to part buttocks from couch and go ahead and actually perform. Countless seminars, books, lectures, tapes, and all manner of other media have been produced on this subject.

As with all of our areas of interest, some of them have merit, some are just junk. Let's have a look at how motivation works and then we'll know who's telling us something worth hearing.

As we examine motivation, let's begin by looking at why we lose motivation in the first place. Think about it. Why do we need to get motivated? Shouldn't we be on fire, all of the time, just chomping at the bit to get out there and take a bite out of life?

It would be nice, wouldn't it? But just like there is Newton's First Law of Motion... A body that is at rest, tends to stay at rest unless acted on by a separate force... there is also Healthy Andy's First Law of Motivation... A butt that sits on the couch, tends to stay on the couch.

Why is that? I've found there's usually two basic reasons why we don't go after what we want. The two patterns that keep us planted firmly butt-to-couch are, simply put, Laziness and Fear.

Laziness we've already discussed. It's the Why Bother pattern, that's all. You remember that one; that's where we give up once we start spinning our wheels. We give, but we don't get. We work, but see no results. So why bother?

We need to conserve energy to stay alive; at least, that's what our bodies are trained through millions of years of evolution to think, and so we hunker down and don't do anything, because that's safer than burning up valuable energy to get nada in return.

Please realize that I call this the Why Bother Pattern rather than the Lazy Pattern for one simple reason. The word 'lazy' carries a lot of negative connotation with it, a lot of emotional baggage.

'Lazy' is bad. Bad, bad, bad. You're a horrible person if you're lazy, and being lazy is always a horrible thing to be.

Not really. Remember, laziness is not a failure of willpower, or some weakness haunting our species. It wouldn't be there if it didn't serve an evolutionary purpose. And the purpose of laziness is, to keep you from burning up valuable energy on frivolous, useless, or counterproductive activity.

We live in a world where you can buy as much gasoline as you want, whenever you want it… so why not drive around constantly? But if a law were passed tomorrow limiting you to only buying three gallons of gasoline a week, you'd be a lot more discriminating with what trips you take with your car!

Running out of gas just means your car stops for a little while, until you can refill it. In your body, it means death. Laziness is a survival mechanism, a throwback to a more harsh time. Unfortunately, in our society, this once-helpful pattern now tends to just get in our way.

And as we've mentioned before, this is an insidious and self-propagating pattern that spirals us down and down into the depths, until we're in a rut we feel we can't get out of. Depression is the extreme end-point of this pattern; giving up on our goals is the first step down the decline.

If you've skipped ahead to this chapter and missed our earlier discussion of this concept, well, big slap on the wrist for you, now go back and read this book in the right order. For the rest of us, we'll just recall what the Why Bother pattern is and why it's there, and move on to Fear.

FEAR: IT'S NOT JUST ABOUT GUYS IN HOCKEY MASKS WITH KNIVES

Fearful living is another pattern, and quite frankly, fear gets a bad rap as far as emotions go. The first thing we think of when we conceive the notion of 'fear' is that of a terrified child, paralyzed with absolutely needless horror at some imagined threat. Or some other image of a weakling laid low by nothing more than shadows on the wall.

Nonsense. Fear works. There's a reason for it to be in our repertoire of emotion: it keeps us alive! While we all like to admire fearless individuals, the truth is, truly fearless individuals often put themselves at foolish risk.

Fear keeps us safe. It keeps us from finding out exactly what happens if we jump off of the roof using an umbrella for a parachute. It keeps us from driving down a busy street at 150 miles per hour (hopefully!). It keeps us from doing the stupid things that make us die young.

We've said before how our bodies are identical physiologically to those of our ancestors running around five or ten thousand years ago. It isn't too hard to understand, given the harsh nature of life in those days, why fear is such a strong and common emotion.

Dangerous situations were a dime a dozen, and in those days, if you were afraid, odds are, you had reason to be. A bad situation nowadays might get you fired. Back in the day, it could get you killed.

Certainly, truly dangerous situations still exist today. But we live in an era of unprecedented personal safety. Our lives are rarely on the line. But our physiology, the natural laws that govern the mechanism that is our body, doesn't know that.

Our physiology doesn't operate on a conscious level. It doesn't 'think' like we do. It just does. It works like a water wheel; automatically, by natural law, without effort. And so we tend to over-use our fear.

While the Why Bother pattern phrase would be "I shouldn't bother because _____________", the Fear pattern phrase would be "I can't because _____________". There's a million possible endings to this phrase.

I can't because, I might lose something precious to me.

I can't because, I might injure myself.

I can't because, someone might laugh at me.

Pick your poison. Notice that some of these phrases might be actually quite sensible reasons not to take action. Some, however, are simply obstacles in our way… which doesn't make them seem any less real or important at the time.

Forget about beating yourself up over being afraid of something; that's nonsense. That's like hating yourself for having to go to the bathroom from time to time. It's just a part of us, a part of being human, so learn to work with it.

The biggest fear that typically holds us back is fear of criticism. Oh, man, is that a big one. To give you an idea of how powerful our fear of criticism is, have a look at this:

MORE PEOPLE ARE AFRAID OF PUBLIC SPEAKING THAN THEY ARE OF DYING!

Isn't that ridiculous? We'd rather die, than get up in front of a crowd and talk about something!

And obviously, there's nothing inherently dangerous about talking to people. Nobody has ever spontaneously burst into flames, or anything like that, based solely on the fact that they were talking to a group. Our fear of public speaking is really a fear of criticism, a fear that we will be ridiculed publicly.

We, as a species, are hard-wired to desire the acceptance of our peers. No doubt this has long-seated roots in our evolution; we are dependent on one another for, well, you name it... safety, specialized services, production of goods we can't make for ourselves, and then, of course, there is the need for social interaction.

No man is an island, goes the phrase, and we all know it to be true. Sure, we'd all like to be less dependent on the opinions of others, but the fact of the matter is, we do care what other people think, we do fear ridicule at the hands of others, so let's not deny that... let's acknowledge it and work with it as best we can.

In the case of these patterns, the Why Bother and Fear patterns, the only way I can think of to deal with them is to disrupt them. We remember seeing how the Why Bother cycle spirals us into depression; the fear pattern spirals us into paralysis. Once again, we have what's called a positive feedback cycle, a loop that feeds on itself, and the trick is to break it… anywhere you can.

Generally speaking, positive feedback cycles are undesirable on a biological level. A commonplace, everyday example of this is something called a **trigger point**, which is a fancy name for a muscle knot.

Injured joints create a structurally unsound situation, which the body controls by tightening up the muscles surrounding the unstable area. This is called **muscle splinting**, and it's what it sounds like… essentially a splint (like the kind you'd use on a broken bone as a first aid device) created by stiffened muscle.

All this is well and good, so long as it's temporary. The problem is, if this unstable situation continues, those tightened muscles get tired. Then they start to hurt, sending pain messages to your nervous system telling it there's something wrong in that area. And then, the body responds by, yes, more muscle splinting. Which then just makes those same tightened, spastic muscles, more spastic. Which makes them more tired, more painful, and so on.

There's actually quite a bit more going on physiologically, but you get the idea. This cycle self-propagates and continues, practically indefinitely, unless it's broken.

Treatment for a trigger point focuses around breaking the cycle anywhere and everywhere you can: by addressing the injured joint, by the use of (sometimes painful) massage to "break up" the trigger point itself, even using injections or electrical impulses to stop the spasm cycle.

So, from one thing, let's learn ten thousand things. Maybe we can't get at the root cause of our fears right away. Maybe we can't change the fact that the Why Bother pattern exists. But we can break the cycle, anywhere we can, in order to disrupt that self-generating pattern and get ourselves moving in the right direction… to get the right patterns firing.

What's the best way to disrupt one of these losing patterns? By succeeding, of course! Which may seem self-evident, but remember, if we do it right, we can halt our decline into apathy, depression, paralysis by fear, you name it, even with a small victory.

There's an old saying I'm fond of…

SUCCESS NEEDS NO APOLOGIES

We're all terrified of criticism. Some of us will go to any lengths to avoid it, even to the point of counterproductive or self-destructive behavior. So we don't even try. We're too afraid. If we never try, we can never fail, if we never fail, well then, nobody can sneer at us and mock our fallibility.

But what if… what if we started off small, perhaps unnoticeable to those around us? Something that might even be considered trivial… like the example of simply drinking water instead of soda at a pizza shop? Then, once we see we can pull that off, we move on, and on, until suddenly, we're ten pounds lighter.

Now we see another part of human nature. Nobody makes fun of a winner… unless they're jealous. Success needs no apologies.

Oh, someone's not impressed that I lost ten pounds by taking slow, almost trivial baby steps? What do I care? I'm ten pounds lighter! Besides, they're probably just jealous because they couldn't do it themselves.

See what I mean? A sense of accomplishment kills fear of criticism. Once we're succeeding, we tend not to care what other people think.

Why? Because we know in our hearts that anyone who tries to tear into somebody simply for being successful is merely jealous. And we're not afraid of jealousy. In fact, on some levels, we like it when other people are jealous of our accomplishments (come on, admit it, you occasionally dig it when a rival grits their teeth and clenches their fists in envy).

Living well really *is* the best revenge. So we don't care if we meet with disapproval, once we're already succeeding.

It's yet another reason to set small, easily attainable goals to create a momentum of success. We've seen already how that defeats the Why Bother pattern of apathy. Now we see that it can also deal with breaking up the paralyzing cycle of the fear of criticism.

What about other fears? Generally, when it comes to achieving goals, if we're not afraid of ridicule, we're afraid that we'll make things worse than they already are.

For example, this would be a common fear if we're just starting to learn how to invest our money. It's a very reasonable concern that if we do something rather than nothing, we might actually lose all of our hard-earned money and end up worse off than before.

Again, the solution is taking little baby steps towards our goal. If we don't commit to a massive level, we can't lose on a massive level, correct? In the example of investing, if we only experiment with a certain investment vehicle and at a small amount… let's say, mutual funds… even if it turns out to be a disaster, at least we're not ruined. And if we see success, we can naturally continue our stepping stone approach forward to a more committed level of involvement.

READY-FIRE-AIM…NOT!

This is why I shake my head at self-help books or gurus advocating rushing at your goals with immediate, complete, utter abandon and disregard for any sort of thought or consideration. "Ready-Fire-Aim", they'll say, or "Just do it."

The idea, of course, is that most of us will feel comfortable studying how to do something, but be too afraid to actually do it. So if you just dive in, now you're moving, and if you're moving, you must be moving forward, right?

Mmm… wrong. The problem with the "Ready-Fire-Aim" approach is, you're gambling. If you miss by being unprepared, and things don't go well at first, you run the very real risk of immediately giving up and falling into one of the losing patterns… either Why Bother or one of the fear patterns.

We've all experienced this in our lives; we get all psyched up about doing something new, making a big change in our lives, and we rush in without thinking, with more energy than sense, and everything goes great until we hit our first roadblock. Then, all of a sudden, the energy disappears. This new change doesn't seem fun anymore. Your goals seem too difficult to achieve. So forget it. Why bother.

It happens every year, usually right after New Year's. Everybody makes their New Year's Resolution to get their sorry butts in shape, and the ranks of health clubs swell with new, enthusiastic, "Ready-Fire-Aim" members who work out two hours a day, every day, for about... oh, two weeks, maybe a month.

Then they get sick of it, and give up, and disappear. "Ready-Fire-Aim", insures you'll miss your mark, and be left with an empty gun.

If, instead of simply rushing headlong into a change of lifestyle, and counting on the initial rush of energy brought on mostly by a sense of novelty, and then hoping willpower will carry them through, if they had paid attention to the natural laws of their bodies, they might have succeeded.

We know that willpower fails; we've discussed it before. Willpower is just our conscious effort in changing an old, natural habit. However, there's a limit to our capacity in this regard, and when stress comes along to slap us in the face... there goes willpower. And then we're right back where we started, because we never formed the new neural network to make the habit we want to form as a natural part of us.

It's easy to get excited about something new, particularly when we have no concept of how difficult it may be to sustain that effort over the long term. Exercise six days a week, two hours every day? Sure! No problem! I'll be buff as a fitness model in no time! Won't that be great!

Sure. Until you actually do it, and the newness fades, and now you're exercising far more than you want to, or are used to, and then that jerk in the cubicle next to you at work doesn't show up, and you're stuck with finishing his presentation on top of your regular work load, and now, all of a sudden, exercise SUCKS, and you don't feel like going. Then your battery dies in your car, and you forget to pay your phone bill, so now you have to deal with that… and before you know it, you practically want to puke when you think of exercise.

It's natural law. You bit off more than you could chew, and when a sudden surge of emotional stress… which as we all know, happens from time to time… comes along, our ability to consciously force ourselves to do something foreign to us goes away. When that happens, we revert back to our natural patterns… the neural networks that have been reinforced the most.

There is only one way to create lasting change in your life. Create a new (or adapt a similar) neural network, and reinforce it until it's second nature.

When we're dealing with fear, particularly fear of criticism, those nice, small, easy stepping stones convince us not only that we're on the right track, but that we can succeed… because we just did!

If we can take one step, we can take another. This new-found confidence increases our faith in the path we've chosen, so if we do have a little stumble, or if it takes a little longer to form and reinforce the new neural network we need to create, we don't freak out and give up.

It allows you to take your time, and keep reinforcing the new pattern, even in the case of a minor setback.

Just like the losing patterns of Why Bother or the various Fear responses, the winning pattern is self-generating as well. Success breeds confidence, which provides motivation, and so long as we follow our simple, realistic, clearly defined goals, stepping-stone by stepping stone, our fitness level will continue to accelerate until we look back at the ground we've covered in amazement.

Could we possibly have traveled so far, so fast? You bet! A pebble can start a landslide, and a loud sound can send an avalanche crashing down the mountain.

From one thing, learn ten thousand things.

To summarize:

- **We start with process-oriented, simple, realistic, and definite goals, broken down into smaller, easier to adapt pieces.**
- **By doing so, we give ourselves more opportunity to recognize that we are actually getting results and not just spinning our wheels.**
- **Concentrating on positive reinforcement is far more effective in the long term than punishment.**
- **Most of us lack motivation through fear or the Why Bother pattern; both are natural, but counterproductive and are most easily disarmed by**

seeing rapid results. Rapid results are most easily
seen with small stepping stones easily achieved in
succession.

CHAPTER 7:

IT'S ALL ABOUT INPUT

We've been talking for a large part of this book about how to create neural networks, habits that will give us what we want in life. But let's not forget the critical first step in the activation of our networks... the specific input.

Remember the knee-jerk reflex? It's built-in, innate; we don't have to practice it or create it. But if your knee's tendon never gets whacked, the reflex will never occur, right? That pattern only fires once a specific input... in this case, stretching the knee tendon... occurs to get it going.

What can we learn from this? Well, we all know that every time a neurological pattern is fired off, or used, it is reinforced. So, the more we get exposed to a certain input, the more likely we are to fire off the corresponding pattern, and the more reinforced that habit will become.

All fitness habits... and fatness habits... are just patterns, neural networks that tend to self-propagate. Whichever patterns you reinforce more, will become more natural. Obviously, then, since we want to reinforce fitness patterns and not fatness patterns, we want to try to favor fitness inputs and avoid fatness inputs.

INPUTS ARE ALL AROUND US

The first source of input I want to talk about is what we see, hear, and smell… what we take in through our senses. Just like the stretch receptors set off the knee-jerk reflex, any of these inputs can activate various patterns related to weight loss.

Here's an example. I used to belong to a gym which was in the same shopping center… in fact, the same building… as a Mexican restaurant. Depending on the time of day, the gym would be filled with all kinds of amazing, appetite-inducing smells.

Not exactly the input you want to take in for an hour or so if you're concentrating on weight loss. The people on the treadmill were practically drooling.

Smells are a particularly powerful stimulus, but don't discount the other senses. Sight is obviously a big one. We are practically inundated on a daily basis with visual inputs designed to make us buy some sort of junk food or another.

As a metaphorical example, imagine some poor sod of a smoker trying to kick the habit who is practically haunted by display ads filled with good looking people smiling and smoking away.

You bet that's an input. So are billboards covered in big ol' burgers, ice cream shakes, slices of pizza, what have you. Even just reading that last sentence might make some people think, "Mmmm… pizza. That sounds *good*."

Ad designers know how to push our buttons, folks. They get
paid to figure out the best way to hit your inputs just right in
order to fire off a pattern so that you buy whatever junk
they're pushing.

It's no wonder we stuff our faces with junk constantly... we
are practically brainwashed on a daily basis by ads designed
to activate patterns of unhealthy eating behavior.

So what can we do about it? Unfortunately, not too much.
The best we can do is try to limit our exposure as much as
possible to those kinds of ads. Avoid places that prominently
display junk food where you can easily grab it. Keep your
blinders on at the grocery store and keep out of the junk food
aisles.

Beyond that, the most you can hope for is to acknowledge the
effects of ads and similar stimuli and recognize that they will
make your job a little harder. Don't attach blame or emotion
to it, simply recognize it and move on.

Now let's talk about an important input system which is
absolutely critical to understand if we not only want to lose
the fat, but lose the fat FOREVER.

Other people.

MONKEY SEE, MONKEY DO

Yep. We're social creatures, folks... no man is an island, and
all that sort of thing... so get used to the idea that those
around you will have a dramatic effect on your neurology.

We know this to be true on an instinctive level; have you ever been sitting next to someone who suddenly yawns, and then you have to yawn as well? "Knock it off!" you say. Sleepiness seems to be contagious.

So does nervousness. Ever have to wait for some important news with someone who won't sit still or shut the heck up? It gets to the point where you want to strangle the little twerp! There you are, trying to keep your cool, and this jerk's emotions keep… well… getting all over you!

Almost every emotion works this way… happiness, sadness, sleepiness, anger, enthusiasm, etc., etc. The people around us act as a source of input for our neurological networks.

We all know we shouldn't "hang out with a bad crowd". Part of that has to do with social psychology, but it also has an important effect on fitness habits.

If you hang out with a bunch of healthy, active people, odds are, you'll end up a healthy person. Hang out with couch potatoes and you'll head in that direction instead.

Misery loves company, doesn't it? Similarly, people encourage those around them to indulge in the same habits they have… good or bad. Unfortunately, most people in this country have horrible health habits, and they seem to like to drag other people down with them.

It's easier to ruin someone else's day than it is to rise above your troubles, isn't it? Then, you would have to admit you have bad habits that need changing, and most people obstinately refuse to do this.

Instead, they would rather see you fail at your attempts at a healthy lifestyle, so they can pat themselves on the back and say to themselves, "See? I knew that was a stupid idea." These kinds of people are literally poison in the well, and must be avoided at all costs.

I see it all the time, folks. Somebody wants to make a positive change in their lives, but their spouse or kids or parents or somebody else that is a major part of their lives sabotages their efforts. Not necessarily on purpose, but if your spouse and kids sit on front of the TV every night with a big bowl of ice cream right in front of you, it's going to make your road a lot tougher.

This point can't be stressed strongly enough. It seems such a simple, self-evident thing, and it fits so perfectly into our neural network theory of fitness that it almost appears we can take it for granted. But really, think about your life, and the people in it. How many of them are boosting you up, and how many are dragging you down?

The problem, of course, is that we can't always jettison those individuals who are troublemakers when it comes to healthy living. Family, co-workers, roommates, there's all kinds of people that we can't really choose whether or not we have to deal with them on a regular basis. So what can we do?

That's a tough one, and there's no easy answer. The first thing I can suggest is, try your very best to limit your exposure to the people sabotaging your efforts, and to increase your exposure to those who boost you up.

Easy for me to say. The other way to do it is to recruit these people into your efforts, make sure they understand that you're trying to make a change and you need their support. There's another possibility as well. Build your own support group, so to speak.

If you can get a few fitness-positive thinkers together to link up, hang out and feed off each other's vibes, you might just be able to pull one of those fitness-negative people out of their slump by having them join in too. By sharing your enthusiasm, your positive energy, you might be able to turn that unhappy sod around and get them on the fitness upswing again… and then, they're not a drain on you at all anymore, are they? Now, they're a positive input, just like you!

Examine carefully the social interactions of fit people. They tend to associate with other fitness-minded, healthy individuals. It isn't just to 'network' in the classic, business-oriented sense (but hey, there's that 'network' word again).

Building a group of friends who all want to stay in good shape, will make it easier for *you* to stay in good shape… because there you are, hanging around the right kind of people, the kind of people who will input into your weight loss, fitness pattern.

HAVING GOOD SUPPORT ISN'T JUST ABOUT YOUR UNDERWEAR

Research shows, over and over again, that the people who are happiest, healthiest, deal with stress the most easily, all that good stuff, are those with a strong social support network. Your support network is a resource whose value cannot be estimated. It quite literally can make or break you.

It doesn't have to be some hokey, corny, silly ritual, with hugging and chanting and banging drums. All it needs to be, is social interaction with the kinds of people you want to be like as much as possible.

There's another part of this equation. Along with negative people, negative *thoughts*, negative actions, and negative words tend to activate the same negative patterns (and, of course, the same is true for the positive end of the spectrum).

Remember how depression is self-generating? Don't sabotage yourself by letting a stray negative thought spiral out of control.

Ever hear the phrase "Whether you think you can or you can't, you're right?" Why do you think that is? Because you're activating whatever pattern corresponds to that input… confidence and enthusiasm inputs to the spiraling up pattern, pessimism and low self-esteem input the fear and Why Bother patterns.

Believe it or not, you have far more control over these stray thoughts than you think. As soon as you can recognize them as simply that (stray little thoughts that have no more meaning than you give them), suddenly their power to influence you decreases.

The next time you have a stray negative thought, like "Exercise is gonna suck today", try to defuse it. Who says it has to suck? It might end up feeling good to get up and move around!

But if you stick to that negative thought, let it bounce around in your mind all morning, you're guaranteed to hate your trip to the gym… it's a self-fulfilling prophecy, thanks to your neural networks.

The words we use are equally important. Try to use words that have a positive connotation, or feeling, to them. My favorite example is "exercise". I try to avoid using the phrase "working out".

Why? Well, look at that second phrase. "Working out". A big part of that phrase is "Work". Who wants to work any more than they have to? You just left work, now you have to go work more? That stinks!

See what I mean? The words we choose can have a subtle effect on us. "Exercise" is neutral, or you might even say has a positive feel.

When I hear "exercise", I think of getting out in the sun, taking the dog for a walk, goofing around in the pool, that sort of thing. When I hear "working out", I think of being tied to an oily, sweat-stained torture device and being forced to beat myself silly.

It may seem silly, or stupid, but it works, and like I said… if it's stupid, and it works, it isn't stupid. The more you can use positive terminology, the more likely you are to react positively to that language.

This goes for so many things in life… the books we read, the movies we watch, so many facets of our life can influence our balance between fitness and fatness by inputting into our neural network.

And I'm not saying you have to obsess over every single one of them… that would be ridiculous. Just be aware of the effect of your surroundings on you. If you find yourself slipping into a fear or Why Bother pattern, seek out some input that will boost you back up… uplifting music, an inspiring book, or fitness-oriented people.

It's critical to control this part of our lives as much as possible. The old phrase "We're judged by the company that we keep" has its roots in this mechanism of other people's influence on our behavior, on activating various parts of our neural networks.

Why do you think so much of what fitness coaches do is essentially jumping up and down and shouting "You can do it!" in one form or another? They're trying to jump-start your motivation and get your momentum going the right way.

So many diet and exercise books are written the same way, filled with more cheerleading than actual real advice or information. This isn't all bad… if it's stupid, but it works, it isn't stupid… as long as you don't need more than a quick burst of inspiration.

Getting back to our social support structure, and our circle of fitness-minded people, the kinds of people we want to be like… can you see how in a way, we're back to hero worship? By socializing with the kinds of people you admire, who are fitness positive, we have the opportunity to expose ourselves to people who might be strong in areas where we are weak.

Maybe you're okay with your diet, but your exercise habits are, well, not so great. If someone in your group is a real exercise nut, I guarantee the more time you spend around that person, the more you'll pick up that 'vibe'… which really isn't a 'vibe', of course, it's just an input into the right neural network in that noggin of yours.

While you're at it, you may start to imitate their behavior, to start forming a new habit or pattern… and here we are, back to Be-Do-Have, back to the beginning of our discussion. Funny how it all links together, isn't it?

IN SUMMARY…

Let's quickly sum up the Mental Game and then see if we can pull it all together for you.

- **We are, in essence, a sum total of the adaptive habits we utilize every day. The more these habits, which are merely neurological patterns, are used, the more they are reinforced and strengthened, until they become second nature… like a reflex.**

- **We can change this behavior using willpower, which is really just our ability to focus on that behavior.**

- **Unfortunately, we have an inborn limit to how much we can focus on at one time. The greater the change (or number of changes) we try to focus on, the greater the strain on this limited resource.**

- **Stress and daily life events also eat up this resource and eventually steal enough that our ability to change our natural, heavily-reinforced habits falls apart. This is when we "fall off the wagon".**

- If we limit the amount of change we attempt to make into smaller pieces, it takes up less of the neurological resource we call willpower, and the more likely it will survive a surge in daily stress. This will allow the new habit to survive long enough to be reinforced, and therefore strengthened, into the new natural pattern.
- By setting goals based on a process, rather than a result, we guarantee a lifestyle change that will last and give us the results we want on a permanent basis. By breaking our large goals down into smaller, more manageable stepping stones, we reduce the strain on our willpower resource, making success more likely.

- This also allows us to see results more quickly, encouraging us to continue and boosting our motivation. In addition, smaller, more manageable goals help to defuse the Why Bother and fear patterns that keep us from trying anything new in the first place.

- By reducing your exposure to negative inputs, whether it be advertisements or people, and increasing your exposure to more fitness-positive inputs, you will encourage the firing of those fitness-positive patterns, which will, in turn, reinforce those patterns, again with the goal of making them eventually become second nature.

SECTION THREE: GO!

CHAPTER 8:
PREPARING FOR THE JOURNEY

In this chapter, we're going to talk all about measuring and the assessment of your waistline. Why? Simple. Because if you're going to map out any journey, you don't just need a destination… you need an origin as well. It doesn't do you any good to know you want to drive to California if you have no idea where the heck you are right now.

There's more to it. As you progress down the road toward your ultimate fitness goals, motivation is going to be critical to success, both in the long-term and the short-term.

That motivation will come from seeing progress, but in order to see progress, you have to get a baseline… a place to start measuring **from**.

What are we going to measure? A couple of different things. For starters, the actual size of the waistline, since after all, this is a fitness book. Obviously we're going to want to see some difference in this area as we go along. Any old tape measure will do.

We also need to get an idea of overall body weight, and in particular, body fat. But it's not as simple as you might want it to be.

HOW FAT IS FAT?

So, let's talk about how fat is fat? The answer, of course, is that there is no definite standard, because any "standard" is by its very nature arbitrary.

However, we can get a notion of vague generalities. The most common, crudest, and most useless way to measure fat versus lean is called **Body Mass Index**, or **BMI** (not to be confused with **BMR**, which is **Basal Metabolic Rate**, a measure of our metabolism…more on this later).

Basically, with BMI, you're dividing your height by your weight. Useless. Why? Well, to use me as an example, even though I'm in pretty decent shape, my BMI calculation lists me as being obese.

The reason for that is simple. I have a lot of muscle mass, more so than average. So while my *fat* content is pretty low, my *weight* is still high, and the BMI calculation doesn't account for that.

There's fudging built in to the equation to account for different "frame sizes", but it's hopelessly crude. Light BMI on fire, toss it in the garbage, and forget it.

The next is **body fat percentage**. This is a far more accurate measurement of what we're really looking to figure out… not if we weigh too much, but if we're too darn fat.

It's what it sounds like… a description of how much fat is on our bodies compared to the rest of us. For men, a range of 8-15 percent is considered healthy or fit. For women, it's more like 18-25 percent.

Men with around nine or ten percent body fat are the guys who start to look "cut", or well-defined; for women, it's around 18-20 percent.

Note that you can go too low with your body fat percentage, and that's just as unhealthy as being overweight. As an example, some competition bodybuilders flex their way up onto stage at about 2-3 percent body fat; and there's been instances where these same guys have dropped dead from that condition… sometimes even during competition!

For women, too low of body fat can interfere with their normal menstrual cycle as well as other health problems. So yes, you really can be "too thin".

The problem with body fat percentage is, it's hard to measure accurately. There's skin-fold caliper tests, which pinch and squish your fat between a set of spring-loaded calipers. These are highly unreliable.

What if one set of calipers squishes more than another? What if the person who is measuring grabs more skin than the last guy? What if he measures at a slightly different spot than the last guy?

It's too difficult to reproduce caliper tests very consistently, so while they're not useless, don't be surprised if several tests come out differently.

There's **bioimpedance**, in which an electrical current goes through you (relax, it's mild enough that you can't feel it) and essentially estimates your body fat percentage based on the resistance of your tissues to that current.

It's a bit more accurate than skin-fold calipers, but you have to follow strict protocols in not eating or drinking beforehand, as water content of body tissues affects the results. For the same reason, measuring yourself at different times of the day may produce different results.

One of the most accurate methods is *water immersion*, in which I dunk you into water and see how much of it you displace. Then I can calculate your density with great precision. The problem is, I need a big giant expensive chunk of equipment to do this, and it's a real pain. So realistically, it and similar high tech methods (like some new advanced X-ray techniques) may not be an option.

Then, of course, there's the good old fashioned way, where we put on our pants and see if they fit, or if we need a shoehorn and a bucket of grease in order to get into them. This is my personal favorite, since it's nice and simple and relates very directly to what we're trying to accomplish (assess our size). You can run into a problem with this, since some clothing manufacturers make their sizes a bit larger than others… and no cheating by using elastic waistbands!

Really, you should be using a tape measure to check the size of your waistline (or other relevant anatomy) accurately. I like to have a pair of "assessment jeans" that I know are the right size so that if they're getting tight, I'm cheating too much on my diet or not keeping up with my workouts. But really, to assess yourself properly, use a tape measure.

Okay, so to answer the question, what should we measure, I suggest using a combination of a couple of things: body weight and certain tape measurements, namely waist, hips, and neck.

The waist tape measurement will give you the most accurate idea of what most people are after: a tight six-pack. But using the other measurements can also give you a good overall idea of how quickly you are shedding those unwanted pounds... and that will inspire and motivate you to continue on.

How big is too big in the waist? For men, if you're over 40 inches, you're getting into the red zone of risk for cardiovascular disease. For women, it's over 35 inches.

There's an interesting calculation created by the US navy to estimate body fat on the basis of height, waist measurement, and neck measurement. It's actually pretty accurate, and easy to perform.

This is the calculation for men: %Fat=495/(1.0324-.19077(log(abdomenneck))+.15456(log(height)))-450

For women, it's: %Fat=495/(1.29579-.35004(log(abdomen+hipneck))+.22100(log(height)))-450

(all measurements are in centimeters)

Or, if you're math challenged like the rest of us, you can just use the online calculator on the US Navy's website:

http://www.mwr.navy.mil/prims/PFAcalculators.htm
(or **http://www.calculator.net/body-fat-calculator.html** if
that one doesn't work)

FOOD DIARY: ASSESS THE MESS

The next thing I recommend that you measure at the
beginning is your dietary habits. You'll soon see that this is
going to be a critical component of getting your way to a
healthier you.

We'll talk a lot about diet in the coming chapters; for now, just
take it on faith that you're going to want to be able to closely
analyze your diet so you can identify areas to improve it.

It's easy to do. Simply write down everything you eat, each
day, for two weeks. That length of time will give you a pretty
good overall idea of what your diet really looks like.

You see, it's too easy to cheat if we just "wing it" and try to re-
create a food diary after the fact. Studies show that
overweight people tend to vastly underestimate how much
they've eaten, and it's just human nature to try to paint
ourselves in the best light possible… even to ourselves.

This is a tricky, insidious part of human nature, my friends.
One of the biggest factors that keep coming up as a problem
in any psychological research study is the tendency of people
to lie on self-report… even if it was anonymous. People don't
like to admit to the negative, even if it's just to themselves…
PARTICULARLY if it's to themselves.

Believe me, when you actually do this, you will be shocked at
what your diet actually looks like on paper. Good. Be

shocked. You need to see this in order to knock yourself into the awareness that a change is necessary.

So do the legwork and keep a food diary for two weeks. And when I say write down everything you eat, I mean **EVERYTHING**. If you eat a Tic-Tac, write down "one Tic-Tac". Drink a glass of water? Write down "one twelve ounce glass of water".

This is the other tricky part. You're going to have to estimate portion size, a classically difficult thing to do. I advise taking a look at an online calorie counter to get an idea of just how big a portion size is. You could always get a small scale and weigh everything, but odds are, you're not going to go to that trouble. I'll be impressed if you actually do the two week food diary at all… most people won't, and that sets them down the wrong path from the beginning.

After all, if you don't know what's wrong, how can you fix it?

I don't want you trying to make any big changes yet. Don't get ahead of yourself. Learn what to do first, **THEN** make your more. In carpentry, they say "measure twice, cut once".

This is what I want you to do. Read through this book in its entirety. If it takes a week, let it take a week. If it takes longer, let it. Read it all the way through so you get an idea of the big picture. Then, go back through it again to sketch out your personal path to healthier habits.

Measure twice, cut once. Don't make yourself work harder by moving before you're ready.

Chapter 9: Diet, Part One

I want you to repeat after me: "Abs are made in the kitchen". Go ahead, say it out loud: "Abs are made in the kitchen". Seriously! Say it for me! It's an old saying in bodybuilding circles, and it's an important concept to drill into your head.

Oh, I know. You **WANT** to just do a couple of crunches or push-ups on the floor and **POOF**! Ready for the cover of a magazine! Sorry, Charlie. Doesn't work that way.

While exercise **IS** important… and we'll cover that subject in more detail later in the book… just as important, if not **MORE** so, is your diet.

Remember, your exercises will shape your muscles, but nobody will ever see them until you burn away the fat layered up over top of them. Diet is the critical component nobody wants to deal with, but I'm here to tell you, it's probably a good 80% of how fat or lean you're going to be.

Okay, there's two basic ideas we're going to go over in the diet chapters. First, is the **quantity** of your food, and second, is the **quality** of your food. Both are important.

Quantity is basically dealing with calories in/calories out, and quality is mostly about the hormonal effects of food on your body. We'll get to that second part in the next chapter, but for now, let's talk calories.

PUT DOWN THE SHOVEL, PICK UP THE SPOON

Controlling the *quantity* of our food is the first step to ridding ourselves of that nasty fat that we're just plain sick of. Portion size is critical, boys and girls; I don't care if you're eating "only good stuff"… if you're eating it with a shovel, you're still going to bust open a few pants buttons.

When it comes to the physiology of weight loss, the main concept you need to understand is, "Calories in, Calories out". You really can't get away from this, no matter what tricks you try to use. Sure, you might be able to bend this law, but you aren't going to break it.

It breaks down like this. Food is a fuel source, which we burn for energy, just like cars burn gasoline. Unlike gasoline, which is a homogenous, consistent substance, we eat all kinds of stuff… chickens, carrots, onions, oranges, bowls of cereal, whatever. All of it gets burned for energy.

 Some fuel sources take longer to burn than others, and therefore we can get more energy out of them. If we have fuel left over that we haven't burned, we store it as fat (mostly) for use later on.

This is all pretty simple stuff that most of us have heard before. Here's a few details to help us quantify what we're talking about. **There are approximately 3500 calories stored in a pound of fat in our bodies.**

That means if you take in 3500 calories of food that you don't burn off, you just added a pound of fat. If you run around like a nut and burn off 3500 calories more than you eat, you lose a pound. That's how it works, simply put. And, simply put, you can't really get away from this, no matter how hard you try.

So how many calories do we use in a day? It's different from person to person. As we all know, some people have "slow metabolisms" and some people have "fast metabolisms". The technical term for our "metabolism" is *Basal Metabolic Rate*, or *BMR* for short. This is an approximation of how many calories you will burn throughout the course of the day, not counting any exercise you put in at the gym… or any other physical activity, for that matter.

Here's how you calculate an approximate value to your BMR:

Women: BMR = 655 + (4.35 x weight in pounds) + (4.7 x height in   inches) - (4.7 x age in years)

Men: BMR = 66 + (6.23 x weight in pounds) + (12.7 x height in inches) - (6.8 x age in year)

If I'm a 170 pound man at 32 years old and 5' 7", my BMR will be about 66 + (6.23 x 170) + (12.7 x 67) – (6.8 x 32)

Which is…

$$66 + (1059) + (851) – (218) = 1758 \text{ calories}$$

So that's how many calories I burn just by being alive and breathing in and out. Then I add in how much energy I burn through my daily activities, which varies wildly, obviously. I don't burn as many calories washing my car as I do running up a hill at top speed.

There's actually a lot of charts out there that will break down how many calories are burned by activity; they aren't really important to our discussion. To give you an idea, though, if you run a mile at an average ten-minute-mile pace, you'll burn off between 100-125 calories, depending on your weight.

More easily, you can estimate about how much your physical activity will add to your energy needs, by using this equation:

- **sedentary** (little or no exercise) : BMR x 1.2

- **lightly active** (light exercise/sports 1-3 days/week) : BMR x 1.375

- **moderately active** (moderate exercise/sports 3-5 days/week) : BMR x 1.55

- **very active** (hard exercise/sports 6-7 days a week) : BMR x 1.725

For a BMR of 1758, the various activity levels break down to these numbers, respectively... 2110, 2418, 2725, and 3032 calories per day.

The point is this. You burn energy two ways... just by being alive, and also by activity. So you can use this to your advantage if you're looking to lose weight by using both of these.

Now that you know about how much energy you burn by lying around, and about how much you burn from your daily activity, you can get a ballpark figure on how many calories you should be taking in to maintain your current weight.

Not that I'm advocating counting calories; in fact, I suggest you don't. It'll drive you nuts in no time flat. Unless you're a competitive bodybuilder or professional model, counting calories takes too much time and effort for you to reasonably expect to keep it up for the rest of your life. And remember, we're interested in forming habits for a lifetime, not the short term.

Still, an occasional look at calorie counts is helpful as a rough gauge as to how much we're taking in… or how much extra we're taking in, as the case may be. If we want to get a handle on portion sizes, it's nice to figure out just how much a "portion" is, isn't it?

Once again, there are charts and charts out there on how many calories are in each chunk of food X, Y, or Z. Or, check the labels on the foods you buy at the grocery store… **and be sure to check what they're calling a portion size.**

You can check the more comprehensive lists out at your convenience. For now, here's a couple listings to give you a rough idea of how a few foods "weigh in":

1 egg……………………………………………..…75 calories
8 oz. Steak…………………………………………… 450 calories
slice of pepperoni pizza…………………….. ..300 calories
medium size apple………………………………..85 calories
12 oz. Beer…………. ………………………………. ..150 calories
medium-sized fast food "combo" meal…….... 1300 calories

ice cream (chocolate).....................300-600 calories/ 1 cup

Are you surprised at some of these?   In particular, are you surprised at how small some of the serving sizes are? At 600 calories a cup, a pint of Ben & Jerry's ice cream clocks in at 1200 calories!

One of the things we find when it comes to overweight people is, they tend to overestimate their activity level and underestimate their food intake. "But I eat right, and I exercise!" they shout, angry and depressed that they're not in the shape they want to be in.

However, if they accurately counted their calories, and measured how much exercise they're really getting, they'd see how the numbers aren't adding up in their favor. This is where calorie counting becomes useful; more as a guide to how much is too much, or too little, but not as a mind-numbing, daily routine.

My advice? Use that food diary you did during your prep stage (last chapter, remember?) and get a rough gauge as to what your caloric intake REALLY is. Then calculate your BMR and daily caloric needs and see if your numbers are adding up for waistline expansion… or contraction.

Here's another tip. When calculating your BMR, use the weight you **WANT TO BE**, not the weight you are right now. After all, we want to know how much fuel you'll need for where you want to be, not where you are.

Chapter 10: Diet, Part Deaux

Now that we have a handle on our *quantity* concerns, let's talk about the *quality* of our food. There's more to it than just calories in, calories out.

Pay close attention to this chapter. This is the missing link that kept me frustrated and angry for YEARS as I struggled to lose those stubborn pounds making my belly jiggle.

Even when I was feeling like I was starving myself, even as I spent five days a week lifting weights and another five running, **STILL** I couldn't lose that fat. Until, finally, **FINALLY**, I came to realize the information I'm about to hand over to you.

Don't struggle uselessly like I did. Or hey, maybe you have already, or are struggling like that now. If you've ever felt like you're killing yourself trying to lose weight, but nothing happens, **READ THIS CHAPTER THROUGHLY**.

You see, the food you eat has effects on your body. Specifically, it can mess with your hormones.

This might sound strange, but we're going to break it down so that it makes perfect sense and you realize the true effects that your diet is having on your body.

First off, we'll talk about carbs and their effect on *insulin*.
Then we'll talk fats and their effect on *cortisol*. Let's get into
it.

THE MUCH-MALIGNED CARB

In the last few years, carbohydrates have gotten a pretty bad
rap. Lots of low-carb diets have popped up, practically
declaring war on anything that even looks like a grain or a
sugar.

Unfortunately, carbohydrates form a significant portion of
those foods dense in micronutrients (vitamins and such), so a
low-carb diet puts us at risk for also being low-vitamin.

Also, most of our dietary fiber comes from carbohydrate-
based foods, and that fiber stuff is what keeps us regular
bathroom-wise (as well as protecting us from ugly stuff like
colon cancer).

So what's the problem? Why are carbs so evil, evil, evil?
Well, they're not… just the way we eat them.

Back in the good old days, the Stone Age, if you wanted to
eat, you either had to forage for food (meaning look for
berries or dig up roots) or hunt (meaning chase something
down and kill it with a pointy stick). So our diets had a mix of
protein, fat, and complex carbohydrates.

But, this method of food collection is, well, unreliable at best.
Maybe berries are out of season, or that pesky deer is just too
quick.

So, somebody came up with agriculture. Now, we had a pile of food, right where we left it. Great, right? Except then we started to process it, to make it last longer in storage.

The problem is this. Your typical carbohydrate has a lot of filler material… fiber and such… which is removed by processing food. What you're left with is closer to being pure carbohydrate… pure sugar, if you like.

The term getting thrown around nowadays is *"glycemic index"*, and it's a concept we want to get a handle on in order to understand why some people hate carbs so passionately.

The idea is this: Since some carbs have a lot of filler material, the body burns it more slowly… if you have a bunch of hay mixed in with a bunch of dirt, it isn't going to burn as easily as just a pure bail of hay. This kind of carbohydrate (the kind with inert filler) has a low glycemic index… it burns slowly.

Pure sugar, on the other hand, burns like jet fuel… it has a high glycemic index. The first problem with sugar is, since it assimilates so easily, you don't get much of a feeling of fullness or satisfaction from eating it. Second, it wrecks all kinds of ridiculous havoc with our *insulin* levels, which is a hormone important to regulating hunger (amongst other things).

In other words, if you eat a handful of cookies, you might've just taken in as many calories (or more) as if you had eaten a steak. But, you won't feel full at all, so you'll just keep on eating, thinking you haven't taken in many calories, and you end up sucking down enough fuel for a dozen lumberjacks without even knowing it.

Let's get back to insulin, which is far more important. When you eat a sugary food… one with a high glycemic index… your body becomes overwhelmed by the sudden spike in blood sugar. In response, it releases a ton of insulin to try to clear that sugar out of the bloodstream.

Why do you care? Because high levels of insulin cause the body to retain fat. It's like a chemical messenger to the body: STORE FAT, NO MATTER WHAT.

With high levels of insulin, your body will store fat, **even if you're calorie deprived**. Instead, it will start breaking down muscle for energy, which really sucks.

If you've starved yourself in the past, and still didn't lose the fat, here's one reason why. If you had ANY refined grains like bread, pasta, crackers, or anything sugary like fruit juice… you spiked your insulin levels and told your body (through that hormone) to store fat no matter what.

Sucks, right? But at least now you know!

There's more to it than that. Insulin acts as an **antagonist** to **Human Growth Hormone** and **glucagon**. A what to what? Let me explain.

An **antagonist hormone** means that it cancels another hormone out or deactivates it. So insulin deactivates Growth Hormone and Glucagon… two important hormones that tell the body to burn fat.

So, not only does it signal the body to **store** fat, it shuts down the messengers that tell the body to **burn** fat (Growth

Hormone also tells the body to build muscle). Talk about a double whammy!

Furthermore, spiking insulin levels makes you feel hungry. Why? Well, because insulin's job is to remove sugar from the bloodstream. So, a huge surge in insulin makes your blood sugar suddenly plummet... the "carb crash" many of you are familiar with. First, the sugar high... then, the sugar low.

When blood sugar levels drop, you feel hunger. When they go into freefall (like after an insulin surge) you get REALLY hungry... especially for more sugar. Since your body is sensing a sudden drop in sugar, that's what it wants.

If it sounds like this system works in a bizarre way with the spiking and dropping stuff, there's a reason for that. Your body isn't designed to process large amounts of refined carbs.

Think of the food available as our bodies evolved. There weren't any Doritos or M&Ms around. There was mostly meat, nuts, fruits, and vegetables. Even though fruit has a lot of sugar in it, it still has a lot of fiber to slow the processing of sugar down... so not so much of an insulin spike (remember glycemic index?).

Nowadays, the processing of food has removed all of the fiber and other stuff that slows the processing of carbs in the body. It's basically been turned into poison.

I'm not kidding. As one medical doctor wrote, "We basically do to our food what we do to cocaine." He's dead right.

Cocaine is actually a rather benign substance in its natural form. It's a green leaf that the local natives chew on slowly, and in this form, it acts as a mild stimulant like coffee. It's only after we take it and refine it… process it… that it becomes super-powerful and addictive.

Sound familiar? Sound like processed foods? It should, because it works exactly the same way.

Okay, I don't want to get up on a soapbox here about the food industry. Let's stick to what you need to know. Summing all this up briefly, sugary foods (or any high glycemic index foods like breads, pasta, etc.) make you get fat.

So it isn't that carbs themselves are bad… just the highly refined, very sugary ones. **Unprocessed** carbs… like vegetables… don't have those bad effects we mentioned earlier. They tend to fill you up a bit longer, and allow your insulin to be secreted at a more steady, reasonable pace.

Seems pretty simple, right? Just avoid sugar! Well, not so fast. The glycemic index is a continuum, so there are some carbohydrates which act so close to the sugar end of the spectrum that might surprise you.

Like pasta, or white bread. These are grains with all or most of the filler (i.e., fiber) taken out, and so they act very much like sugary type foods when ingested.

Why do we eat those refined carbohydrates at all? Simply put, they are the easiest fuel source to grow in abundance. Remember, for most of the history of our species, the problem wasn't how to stay thin. It was how to avoid starvation.

So we came up with a reliable, easy, cheap source of energy… grains. And, to help preserve them longer and make them taste better, we started refining them, never realizing that we were taking out vital components of our food. We traded healthy food, for cheap, easy, and abundant food.

Unprocessed foods are more expensive. Do a cost comparison at the grocery store between canned or refined food, and whole, organic fruits and vegetables. The price difference can be considerable. Of course, my feeling is, the extra expense is worth it. Nothing is more valuable than your health.

My suggestion when it comes to carbohydrates is this: first off, limit the amount of processed carbs you take in, whether it be cakes, pastries, and candy, or pastas, refined breads, and the like. It's tricky to do so, trust me, because they sneak into a lot of our foods.

But the more you can cut refined carbs (or refined foods of any kind), the faster the fat will fall off of your abs. Stress fruits and vegetables (not juice, that's just sugar water) in their natural state.

Also, for me, I find that it works best to eat more carbs earlier in the day, and taper off until evening, when I eat very little carbs. The reason for this is simple. Carbs are our immediate power source.

So, I need them when I'm running around, doing things actively. But, at night, I'm usually not very active… in fact, I'm asleep for a good eight hours of it. So I don't really need a lot of immediate energy, do I? And remember, any excess energy that doesn't get used right away, gets stored as fat.

In addition, get rid of soda. It's just sugar water and chemicals you don't want in you. While you're at it, watch out for **high-fructose corn syrup**, which is a super-sugary sweeter that's far worse for you than just eating a handful of sugar. It's all over the place, too… look through a couple of food labels and I think you'll be surprised how many processed foods have this junk stuck in there.

THE MUCH-MALIGNED FAT

Here's another macronutrient that gets a worse reputation than it deserves. Once again, fat isn't bad all by itself; it's how we ingest it that creates a problem.

Fat is a very calorie-dense fuel source; while proteins and carbs give us about four calories per gram or so, fats give us nine calories per gram. Now, in today's world, we shriek and run in horror at the idea of a calorie-dense food. But back in the day, getting a fatty meal was a bonanza, a windfall of life-giving energy that could sustain us through some pretty tough times.

So it's not a real surprise that our bodies crave fatty foods. They helped us survive back in the day. But it goes beyond that.

Fats help us build certain vital tissues in our bodies as well… the membranes that make up the cellular walls of our bodies, for example. More in line with our discussion on losing body fat to unleash our inner six-pack, fats also tend to give us a more satisfied, full feeling after we eat them. Also, because high-fat meals move more slowly out of the stomach than low-fat meals, we also feel fuller, longer.

The problem occurs, of course, when we go overboard and no longer consume fat in moderation. Some fat is vital to our health, but if we're chowing down on bowls of lard, well, we can all guess how that's not so good for us.

There's another way in which fats can affect our lives... the hormonal effects of fat intake. Lately, a major hot topic in health care research is the importance of **inflammation** in the various tissues of the body; in particular, the effects of long-term, chronic inflammation.

In fact, lots of white-lab-coat-types studying heart disease are starting to stray away from using cholesterol levels as the best indicator of cardiovascular disease, claiming that chronic, low-level inflammation is far more important to keep an eye on.

What does this have to do with losing body fat? Well, for purposes of our discussion, there's basically two kinds of essential fatty acids (fats you actually need for your body): Omega-3 and Omega-6 Fatty Acids.

Sounds like a Star Trek term, right? But take the time to learn the difference, because it has huge long-term consequences to your waistline. The names come from the difference in molecular structure of each fatty acid; namely, the location of the first carbon double bond. That's not important.

Here's what is important. Omega-3 fatty acids tend to **decrease** inflammation, while Omega-6's tend to **increase** inflammation. How and why is complicated; it has to do with each being a biochemical precursor to different substances in the body. The details, again, are not important to this discussion.

While both Omega-3 and Omega-6 fatty acids are essential to our diet, unfortunately, the advent of processed foods and grain-fed agriculture has led to a massive imbalance in our ratio of these fats. We should have a one to one ratio; equal parts Omega-3 and Omega–6. But we don't.

 Some estimates are that our diets are skewed as much as twenty to one in favor of Omega-6s, the "bad" fats that cause inflammation. **Twenty to one!**

Why are we eating so many Omega-6s? For the same reason we eat lots of refined carbohydrates: they're cheaper. Specifically, they have a longer shelf life, and are easier to use in certain kinds of foods, than Omega-3s.

And, we feed it to our livestock, in the form of corn (which is high in Omega-6s). Since the livestock eats lots of Omega-6s, they're full of Omega-6s when we get around to eating them.

Grass-fed livestock, on the other hand, have a much more balanced fat profile (including eggs produced by grass-fed hens). But grass-feeding is expensive, so, most livestock are fed corn or other Omega-6 heavy grains.

Also, when you refine a fat, you alter its molecular shape to turn it into an Omega-6, or worse, a "trans" fat. Fried foods are fried in Omega-6 fats; you're basically soaking your food in this pro-inflammatory substance.

All of these factors add together to create that massive twenty to one imbalance which is making our bodies exceptionally prone to inflammation.

We can all see why this is a problem health-wise, but what does that have to do with your weight? Simple.

Inflammation is linked to a stress hormone called *cortisol*, and cortisol makes our bodies deposit fat around our bellies (in a similar way to insulin). In fact, some doctors refer to belly fat as a danger sign for heart disease, because belly fat means cortisol, cortisol means inflammation, and inflammation means heart disease.

This is not a book about heart disease. But, it is a book about weight loss, and most of us would like to lose that belly fat that's been annoying the crap out of us, right?

So if we reduce our Omega-6s, and increase our Omega-3s, we can promote loss of fat in that area by reducing the amount of inflammation going on in our bodies.

We find omega-3's in stuff like fish, walnuts, and green leafy vegetables. You can also supplement with fish oil or flaxseed oil. Since I don't like to eat fish, I use supplements to get the Omega-3's that I need.

The bottom line is, don't run screaming from fats just because they're called "fats" and you don't want your friends to call you the same thing. Fats are a crucial part of our diet, critical to our health, and if used in moderation, will actually make your weight loss easier (by making you feel fuller, longer)… so long as you use them in moderation, of course!

Again, the key is to avoid processed foods. When it comes to animal products like eggs and meat, look for "free range" and "grass fed" on the label. This means that the chicken or turkey or cow was raised out in a field, eating grass the way they're meant to, rather than being cooped up in a cage and eating nothing but Omega-6 filled grains.

The last thing to mention when it comes to discussing fats is the horrible, horrible "trans fats". You've probably heard this term.

Basically, a trans fat is a man-made fat. As you might imagine, that means we aren't going to want to eat it.

These are fats that have been modified to last longer or simulate certain textures or flavors. The short answer is, they're poison. Plain and simple. Think of them like Omega-6 fats, but worse.

And, of course, there's tons of them in processed foods… margarine especially. Avoid this stuff like the plague, and stick to healthy fats, like olive or coconut oil.

CHAPTER 11:
DIET, MADE EASY

All of this talk about calorie counting and hormonal effects of different foods can make your head spin after a while. I get it. So, don't get too caught up in it.

Seriously. Counting calories, reading ingredients on each and every scrap of food you eat… who's going to keep up with that? I mean, who's going to keep up with that, **for a lifetime**?

Oh, sure, you might do it for a week or two, but what happens when the poop hits the fan at work and you have to pull double shifts, or the kids burn the back yard down, or some other Disaster Of Life strikes (which you know it eventually will)? What then?

Or what happens when you just plain get sick of trying to keep track of all these stupid diet details? You'll give up, is the answer. Of course you will. Anybody would. It's human nature.

So stop trying to fight human nature. Keep things simple.
I'm a huge fan of simple. My life is enough of a whirlwind; I
don't need a bunch of EXTRA details to keep track of on a
daily basis. So, let me give you a simple all-around strategy
that will take care of all of the diet details automatically.

THE EASY ANSWER

For those of you who just want to cut to the chase and get the
quicko-easy answer, here's one way you can be sure to limit
your caloric intake, keep your glycemic index low, and deal
with your good and bad fats. **Eat whole foods.**

That's it?

Yeah, pretty much. It's a simple sentence, but trust me, folks,
it ain't easy. Don't believe me? Take a walk around your
local grocery store and pick out which foods are actually
whole, unrefined foods. You'll skip about eighty percent of
the store. Maybe more.

In fact, our food supply is so highly processed, it can be hard
to tell what is a whole food in the first place! I used to joke
with my patients, if you can pick it off of a tree or kill it with a
stick, it's a whole food.

WHOLE FOODS DEFINED

Raw fruits and vegetables, eggs, meats, nuts… these are all
whole foods. Some people add whole grains into that
group… I would suggest limiting them.

You might need a little oatmeal or rice or something similar to help add a little fiber to your diet, but most grains aren't anywhere near as nutrient dense as fruits and vegetables, and it can be tricky sometimes to make sure your grains haven't been refined at all.

The only people I think really need grains are athletes or individuals whose jobs are very physically active. For these people, it's unlikely they can get enough calories in to keep up the necessary performance level without some rice or oatmeal adding some calories in to the mix.

Odds are, though, you don't need them. So avoid grains if you possibly can… the more you avoid them, the faster you'll drop the weight you don't want.

Notice that "pasta", "bread", "cereal", and "canned fruits or vegetables" are not on the list of whole foods. Neither is "soda" or "Fruit juice"; remember most fruit juice is really sugar water with artificial juice flavor added. If you want to squeeze your own juice at home out of fresh fruits and vegetables, that's another matter. But skip the sugar water.

And "meat" doesn't mean "pepperoni" or "sausage" or "bacon". These are all *processed* meats. Meat means… steak, chicken breasts, fish (not fried!), turkey… you get the picture.

And if you fry a turkey in one of those huge turkey fryers on Thanksgiving, guess what. Not a whole food anymore. You just fried it, and soaked it in Omega-6 fatty acids. Fried foods of any kind are NOT whole foods.

Still confused? Let's have a list of some examples of whole foods and not whole foods:

WHOLE FOODS	NOT WHOLE FOODS
Apple	Apple juice, apple pie
Steak	Hamburger Helper
Chicken Breast	Microwave Chicken Dinner
Peach	Canned Peaches
Oatmeal	Oat bread/ Oat flour
Tomato	Ketchup, Tomato sauce
Carrot	Carrot Cake
Corn (on the cob)	Corn chips, corn bread

Are we starting to see the trend here? Any modification of the food from its natural state makes it not a whole food. The more you modify or change a food, the less healthy it becomes.

Another rule of thumb: if it comes in a box or a can, you don't want it. So much junk gets added to these kinds of foods, that even if they LOOK okay, they're filled with salt and sugar and MSG and God Only Knows what other crap that will make you fat and eventually kill you.

Doesn't sound so simple any more, does it? But here's the good news. By avoiding processed foods, you will automatically control your glycemic index (and therefore insulin) without having to look up or calculate any sorts of values.

You will also control your caloric intake, so long as you don't absolutely stuff yourself. Why? Because now that you're not sucking down gobs of empty calories, and you are eating fiber and good fats and proteins and low-glycemic foods instead, you will feel full when you should feel full.

Remember, with sugar, you can fire down as much of that stuff as you want and never feel full. When you start eating real, whole, unprocessed foods, you're going to feel full when you've had enough.

Of course, if you eat until you feel stuffed, you're shooting yourself in the foot. Take your time as you eat. Don't eat until you are stuffed, but until you are simply no longer hungry, and the calories will count themselves.

The funny thing is, as you get more and more used to a whole foods diet, you'll wonder why you never ate that way in the first place. We're so bombarded by TV and magazine ads for quick, easy, refined foods, that we forget how good whole foods taste and make us feel.

And you know what? Whole foods are pretty darn convenient too. You don't have to do much to a carrot or apple or almond in order to make it ready to eat. We're talking near-zero prep time!

Of course, you're still going to want your occasional burger or slice of pizza or hunk of ice cream. That's fine. We're going to talk next about how to transition into a whole foods diet without going insane, starving ourselves, or giving up our occasional indulgences.

HOW TO GET FROM HERE TO THERE

In this section, we're going to start by going over how to transition from a Fatness diet habit of processed and junk foods into a Fitness diet of whole foods, and in such a way that you won't hate your life.

Then, we'll talk about how to cheat PROPERLY, so you can have your indulgences and also avoid climbing a bell tower with a high-powered rifle due to lack of chocolate.

We're going to start off with a discussion on our patterns of behavior. After all, that's all "diet" means, is a particular pattern or habitual way of eating. Which means you're already on a diet, whether you know it or not.

I'm sure it's also no shock when the first thing I have to say about diet… and in particular, changing our diet… is, **forget any kind of fad diet**. Burn whatever book you read that fad diet in, hit the embers with a rock, and throw the ashes out of the window.

Please note that I define a "fad diet" as **any diet that is not designed to be used for the rest of a person's life**… whether the inventor claims it can be or not. And while there's a gray area when it comes to this sort of thing, we all have a pretty good idea of what we can keep up for the rest of our lives.

Here's why any ridiculous, unrealistic fad diet is doomed to failure. Quite simply, it's unnatural… to us, at least. Our dietary habits are just that, habits, patterns, a neurological network reinforced several times every day, both through repetition and the positive reward we get from pleasurable eating.

Now along comes Dr. So-and-So with his Amazing Breakthrough Diet. Lose a hundred pounds in six days, guaranteed! All you have to do is, focus your entire daily life with examining, planning, and preparing your food intake in excruciating detail, and make yourself miserable daily by forcing all kinds of crap down your throat that you want nothing to do with!

Riiiight. That'll work. Sure. That's why we have an epidemic of obesity in this country (and frankly, it is an epidemic). I wonder why that is? I can assure you it's not for a lack of fad diets.

Let's start with the fallacy of a "Breakthrough" diet. Don't forget that our bodies operate under the same natural laws as the ancient Greeks, Romans, Indians, Chinese, and everybody else… do you really think that during the last 5,000 years, not one person figured out healthy eating habits?

Granted, they may not have had the level of scientific knowledge that we do when it comes to nutrition, but they had fat people and thin people and professional athletes and idle couch potatoes and all the same stuff as we do. We have two things the ancient world lacked, when it comes to food.

One, is abundance.

Two, is highly processed food.

We've already discussed both of those concepts in detail, so you can just scrap the notion that there's any amazing dietary breakthroughs, anywhere. Our bodies haven't changed for thousands upon thousands of years; what's changed is what we stuff into them.

An unusual fad diet regimen might suggest that some "secret" has been unlocked, one that has been overlooked for the last

5,000 years by every single person who has ever lived. Folks, there's no such thing. We all know it.

But, our curiosities are piqued by the unusual, and the mysterious, and fad diet proponents prey on that by concocting ridiculous draconian regimes that will provide exactly jack squat in the long term.

How do I know this? Look at the phenomenon of yo-yo dieting. That's when someone goes on "a new diet", loses a bazillion pounds, then two, three, or maybe six months later, freaks out, eats seventeen thousand buffalo wings in one sitting, and balloons back out to their previous weight (or worse). Then, they find another diet, and repeat the process, yo-yo up, yo-yo down, back up, back down, and so on.

JUST SAY NO TO THE YO-YO

Forcing ourselves to follow a new weird diet requires a great deal of conscious effort… we call it "willpower"… because we're fighting an incredibly powerful (strongly reinforced) neurological pattern… our old diet habits. Not only are we resisting our natural habit, we're making massive changes to that habit, all of which requires that pesky, unreliable willpower stuff to make it stick.

So, at first with this new diet, we lose some weight, and we're encouraged by that, so we chug on, forcing ourselves to eat nothing but… grapefruit, oat bran, bags of grass clippings, whatever… no matter how much we hate it. And a feeble, unreliable new habit starts to form.

Then, we blow a tire on our way to work, right in the middle of a rainstorm. On the same day, mind you, as the school calls to tell us our beautiful youngest child just bit somebody's nose during recess, and the septic tank explodes in the back yard, showering your lawn with a sort of fertilizer that you didn't plan on.

In a flash, we're down at Fat Charlies's Rib Shack, sucking down chicken wings like it's our job. Here's what's happened. Stress overwhelmed our cognitive capacity to modulate our neurological patterns (that's what we call "willpower") and, following natural law, we reverted back to our old habits, our patterns hard-wired into our bodies through constant, daily reinforcement throughout our entire lives.

And then, of course, we throw up our hands in disgust at our failure, as weak, pitiful creatures, and in our misery, we stop at the Old Time Ice Cream Depot on our way home to down two banana splits to drown our sorrows, as we spiral down into despair (I call it the Why Bother neurological pattern) and give up.

Several things happened here to doom us to failure. First off, we fought against not just our habits, but natural instincts. Never forget that **we're not designed for a modern life of plenty**; our bodies were forged to survive in a harsh existence where life was much more famine than feast.

Our bodies are naturally inclined to want to binge on all kinds of fatty foods, sugary stuff, you name it, as much as possible, to protect us against lean times. So if we push our bodies too far and jump into an extremely restrictive diet, you can count on your body making you miserable until you give in.

Perhaps I shouldn't say that our bodies make us miserable; that implies a conscious effort to punish ourselves. Try to remember that the natural laws of our body are not good or bad… they just are.

Pain, naturally, has a negative connotation or feeling attached to it. It had better! It's a signal designed to make us avoid what's hurting us. Without pain, we'd tear ourselves to pieces, which is exactly what happens in certain neurological conditions… the patient can't feel that they are hurting themselves, and they literally tear themselves apart.

Hunger is a similar signal. It feels nasty, doesn't it? It had better feel nasty! It's like pain; a signal that the fuel tank is getting low, and we need to load up.

But again, like pain, it's neither good or bad… it just is. How we deal with it determines its value. So when I say the body will make us miserable if we fight our natural desires, what I mean is, the body is geared toward certain things… like feasting when the feasting is good… and when we starve ourselves, we're going to get some uncomfortable signals from our bodies.

Our bodies don't understand that we want to fit into a size 6 dress in time for that wedding that is rapidly approaching, or that summer is coming and we need to get washboard abs pronto. Our bodies don't "think" on a cognitive level. They work as best suits our survival, and for most of our existence, that meant survival in lean times.

Getting back on track, remember that our dietary habits are patterns of behavior that are being reinforced every day, several times a day, and not just through repetition.

There are other pleasure-pathway reward mechanisms at work here; in fact, there's research showing that sugar is more addictive than cocaine, and that junk food activates the same neurochemical reward pathways in the brain as heroin and opium! So the influences we're trying to fight are incredibly strong, and here we are trying to wrestle it to the ground as if we were grabbing a bull by the horns.

I have news for you. If you go grab a bull by the horns, you're going to end up gored and stomped into the dirt. There are better ways to handle dealing with a powerful, ingrained pattern of behavior, and head-on isn't one of them.

It's too much of a change, too far, too fast, too much, and that means we have to dedicate a tremendous amount of mental effort (willpower) to maintain that change.

And there's the problem. We relied on willpower alone, pure bull-headed stubbornness, to get us through, when that never works long-term. Sure, if the only thing we had to worry about every day was planning and preparing our super-restrictive diet, then we might pull it off.

But life is a bit more chaotic than that, and we usually have to deal with a lot of crap that jumps out of nowhere and slaps us in the face. That uses up our mental energy as well, and when that runs out....

...pull up a chair at Fat Charlie's. Basically, we just jumped into the ocean and said "I'll just keep swimming, and if I get tired, why, I'll just keep on going, no matter what." Riiiiiight. 'Cause THAT'S a good idea.

People get tired, ladies and gentlemen; that's just the way it is. We're not robots. We get tired, we get overwhelmed, we get sick of the struggle, and when that happens, we go back to what's easy to us… what's natural to us.

And so, because of all these mistakes, we reverted back to our natural habits once our willpower ran out, as it always does. Once we failed our lofty, over-ambitious goal, the tendency to blame ourselves for not being perfect kicked in, and then we labeled ourselves a loser and gave up.

I realize this sounds awfully gloomy, but it really isn't. We're just examining the mechanics of what goes wrong with the vast majority of dieting… and now that we know what goes wrong, and why it goes wrong, we can fix it. First off, we don't give in to fad dieting, no matter how tempting those quickie results might sound. Remember, easy come, easy go, especially when it comes to lifestyle change.

FAT LOSS FOREVER

So how do we make a major change in our eating habits, when we've been used to eating this way our entire lives? And how do we do it without blowing ourselves out of the water with stress? We get there by using stepping stones.

This is what it sounds like… breaking down our long-term goal into smaller, easier pieces. There's an old saying that goes like this: "How do you eat an elephant? One bite at a time."

That's what we're going to do. It's insane to think that someone who's been hooked on junk food, convenience food, high carb food, or whatever that person might be used to, is going to just stop instantly and make a 180 degree turn in behavior, permanently. It just doesn't work that way.

And if you pile up too much on your plate (metaphorically speaking), the odds go up dramatically that you will overwhelm yourself with too much change, too fast. Back in the section on The Mental Game, we discussed how human beings have limits as to how much change they can really handle at any particular time.

Some people want to think they can handle anything, any time, and anything less is just being a sissy. I call these people "doomed for failure". They're the ones who take off sprinting at the beginning of a marathon, and you find them a mile into the race keeled over on the side of the road, puking.

We're about to see exactly how we're going to use this concept to fix our diet, but first, there's one more thing to discuss: how to indulge, without adding to your bulge.

LEARNING TO BREAK THE RULES PROPERLY

When it comes to habits like diets, the patterns are usually so strong that we can't completely eradicate them… at least, not for a few years. The reason is simple; we're constantly bombarded by stimulus that inputs into those patterns… think TV ads for fast food or candy or whatever.

Or how about holidays like Halloween or Easter, chock full o' candy? Or parties, happy hours, or other social engagements where we're encouraged to eat exactly the way we're trying not to?

All of these are inputs, which activate that habit we're trying to get rid of… eating too much junk.

Simply put, odds are, very few people will be able to quit eating junk food entirely. And so what? An occasional burger isn't going to make you keel over, dead, dead, dead, right on the spot. Nor is it going to make you instantly blow out to three hundred pounds. An occasional "cheat" is fine; in fact, it's what will keep you sane!

The trick is, not to let those "cheats" get out of hand. And the easiest way to do that is to **quantify in a specific way** how much you'll let yourself cheat.

For example… some of the best advice I ever got, as far as controlling my diet goes, came from a bodybuilder I met while I was working my way through school in a coffee shop.

This guy was about forty years old, and looked more like twenty-five. To say he was buff would be a ridiculous understatement… the man was chiseled like a Greek statue.

And yet, every Sunday, he'd come rolling into the coffee shop, and buy every cookie, brownie, whatever you can think of, that we had!

Curiosity got the better of me one day, as it often does, and I had to ask him just what the heck was going on. How did he stay in such incredible shape while firing down all those sweets?

His answer was, it was his cheat day. All week, every week, Monday through Saturday, he watched his diet with microscopic precision: chicken breasts and broccoli for dinner, tuna and brown rice for lunch, that sort of thing. But come Sunday, the reins were let slip, and he allowed himself to eat anything he wanted, and as much as he wanted.

Brilliant.

Let's be honest. Who's giving up chocolate for the rest of their lives? I don't think so. And how many of us are going to really give up that handful of delicious somethings that we know are bad for us, but taste so darn good… forever?

Forget it! It's unrealistic for us to expect our willpower to hold us off from that stuff our entire lives.

And, quite frankly, who the heck wants to? If being built like a fitness model means never eating ice cream for the rest of my life, then forget about seeing my bod on the cover of any magazines!

Life's too short to completely deny ourselves ANY fun, ANY indulgences… let's just keep them in check, shall we?

Here was a guy who found a way that he could indulge periodically in what he wanted, and still maintain an outstanding physique. I can't swear off of eating a slice of pizza ever again; but I CAN hold off for a few days if a craving strikes.

That's reasonable. So I hold out for my Cheat Day. Another reason for a Cheat Day is as follows.

Remember those hormonal effects of foods? Well, it just seems to work better if you keep from having any insulin or cortisol surges for days at a time, rather than have a little surge every day.

So, if you have to splurge, it's better to splurge just once in a big way than many times in a little way. So don't cheat a little each night; set aside a day once a week… your Cheat Day.

Or Cheat Weekend, if you like. After all, if you're not shooting for a bodybuilder's physique, your controls don't need to be quite as tight. Just don't let it be a Cheat Six Day Weekend!

See what I mean? We've quantified our little cheats; we've put a definitive rule on them and so now we can keep accurate track of them, hold them to a certain limit.

PUTTING IT ALL TOGETHER

So here's how we do it when it comes to diet. We're going to slowly change over our diet habits, from processed junk Fatness Foods, to unprocessed Fitness Foods. We're going to do it one day at a time in little stepping stones.

We then reinforce those individual stepping stones thoroughly before we move on to the next. That way, if we do stumble, we don't go all the way back to the beginning, like a game of Chutes and Ladders. It's sort of like saving your progress on a computer; if there's a crash, you won't lose it all.

The eventual goal is to eat all whole foods, six days a week, and then have a Cheat Day for your indulgences. That's the destination.

Where you are today is the start, obviously. If you're eating junk food every day, start by cutting out one day during the week during which you'll eat only healthy foods... I suggest Monday.

So, on Monday, it's nothing but healthy, unprocessed foods, heavy on the fruits and vegetables. Drink nothing but water. A one hundred percent, no cheats, whole foods diet day.

The day after that, you go right back to what you're used to. However you normally eat, that's how you eat, Tuesday through Sunday.

Sounds easy, right? Maybe too easy? It should sound easy. It's SUPPOSED to be easy. This is just the first step, designed to get you going in the right direction and simultaneously show you that a whole foods diet really isn't such a big deal.

After a few Mondays of this, add Tuesday. Again, every other day, eat as you normally would, but Monday and Tuesday, you eat one hundred percent, all whole foods, NO EXCEPTIONS.

Actually, a lot of you are going to be able to start at two days a week (Monday and Tuesday) of whole foods. It's really very easy, especially when you know that come Wednesday, you can go right back to what you're used to.

I mean, really, once you do it once or twice, you're going to say to yourself, "Why did I think this was going to be a big deal?". I know that's what I said.

Once you feel like two days a week is too easy…and ONLY then… you add Wednesday to the whole foods day list. And so on, and so forth, until you've stepping-stoned your way to only eating your indulgences on the weekend… and then finally just one day a week.

It's a long process, but it's the only way to really insure that A) you don't push yourself too far, too fast and fall off of the wagon and B) that you KEEP these fitness habits (and therefore, your fitness body) for a lifetime.

What if you DO feel overwhelmed? Say you just added the fourth whole foods day, and then you have a Week From Hell and are ready to burn the entire city down to the ground. And you freak out and have a cheat day on Thursday when you wanted to have a whole foods day.

No problem. Go back to three days a week of whole foods, and stay there until you feel like it's easy again. It's no big deal. You're trying to change a habit that's been hammered into your mind for DECADES; it's not going to go away overnight.

Soon enough, you'll be comfortable with those three days of whole foods again and ready to move on to four days once more. And so on and so forth, until you get to six days of whole foods, and one Cheat Day.

And on that Cheat Day… LIVE IT UP! I mean it! Go crazy on whatever you've been craving. You might even feel a little sick by the time you're done… GOOD. That will just make it all the more easy to go back to whole foods the next day!

Believe it or not, eventually, you will come out of your Cheat Day(s) looking FORWARD to healthy whole foods. I know I do. Cheat Day makes me feel like crap… not emotionally, but physically. I can really feel the effects of the sugar and junk. I get sluggish. My body swells up, retaining water from the sugar. I basically just feel awful. All that reverses pretty quickly come Monday and my return to a whole foods diet.

You're going to notice the same thing once your body starts feeling good from all that healthy food. You'll feel better when you're eating them, and the fat starts disappearing from body, you'll be loving whole foods even more!

Congratulations! You've learned everything you need to know about diet to get yourself lean for a lifetime. Pat yourself on the back for this milestone; **you now know more about diet than about 90% of personal trainers** (particularly the mental part).

And, the sooner you start implementing this gradual shift over from fatness foods to fitness foods, the sooner you're going to get your body to look exactly the way you want it to.

CHAPTER 12:
EXERCISE PART ONE: AB EXERCISES

Let's talk about the area of the body that everybody screws up. It's also the spot we all want to look good… the waistline.

We used to refer to this area as our "abs", but that's kind of a misnomer. The abdomen is the front half of your body, and as we've come to learn over the years, it's important to exercise and develop the *entire* ring of muscles that sheathe your midsection… front, back, and sides.

I see four basic errors when it comes to training the midsection… and the first is, when people simply don't do it at all. For some reason, people hate to "do abs", or whatever else you want to call it. I'm one of them. So let's start with why this muscle group is so darn important.

It's not the reason most people think, which is "look really hot with your shirt off". But I'm getting ahead of myself. The main reason you need a strong midsection is to *avoid injury*. You see, the muscles of the trunk act like a ring that compresses the abdominal contents to protect the joints of the spine.

Think of it like a weight belt. Most of you have seen a weight belt… either on an Olympic powerlifter, or on somebody working at Walmart who has to lift things all day, or on somebody *somewhere*. It's a big wide belt that goes around the belly and low back, and it works by compression.

By compressing that area, you increase the amount of stabilization around the spine, thereby protecting the joints from any sudden shearing forces they might encounter as you strain at lifting a heavy weight until the veins bulge out on your head.

The muscles of your midsection act like a built-in weight belt. By squeezing inwards in a ring, they stabilize the spine and keep those delicate joints from getting torn by whatever crazy shenanigans you're up to that day. They also support the internal organs and keep them from falling out of our belly, but hey, that's hardly important, right?

The point is, you need to keep the muscles of your midsection healthy and toned, and not just for purposes of vanity. Let's talk about that, next.

OUT, DAMNED SPOT!

Repeat after me. *There is no such thing as spot reduction of fat.* Louder. *THERE IS NO SUCH THING AS SPOT REDUCTION OF FAT.* Again. AGAIN! Shout it!

The myth of spot reduction of fat…somehow removing fat from one area of your body rather than another… has been unbelievably persistent over the years. Doing endless crunches to get a "six-pack" set of abs does about as much good as my all-time favorite Quack-O nonsense exercise machine… that big fabric belt that goes around your love handles and vibrates. I LOVE that thing. Yeah! SHAKE the fat off! *That'll* work!

One more time, folks. *There is no such thing as spot reduction of fat.* Forget it. It's a lie. You lose fat all over your body, or not at all. If you want a skinny waist, you have to lose fat all over, including your waist. That's how it works. Sorry.

Having a toned set of muscles can keep your midsection a bit thinner as the tape measures, since those toned muscles will be less apt to bulge out from the strain of holding your guts in after you splurge on those extra couple of burritos, but it won't do anything about the layers of fat laying on top of those muscles (which is what determines muscle definition, or how well you can see the striations of the muscle).

Think of your body like a cake. Just like you have a layer of icing on top of the cake, you have a layer of fat laying on top of your muscle (and just beneath your skin). It doesn't matter how dense the cake itself is; if you heap tons of icing on top of it, you'll never see the cake part. You have to scrape the icing off.

That's how you get muscle definition. Fat loss. And you lose fat globally, all over, in a pattern largely determined by gender and genetics. It sucks, yes, but that's how it works. The only way to spot reduce fat is surgically (liposuction), and that has its own set of complications that are beyond the scope of this book. Bottom line; forget spot reduction. It doesn't happen.

DON'T JUST BE CAPTAIN CRUNCH; THERE'S A BACK AND SIDES AS WELL

The next big mistake people make is "doing abs" by just "doing crunches". The crunch, for those of you not in the know, is the 21st Century version of the sit-up. Basically it's a sit-up without your feet planted under anything. The point is, it's an exercise for the rectus abdominus muscle… the so-called "six pack", or ribbed section of muscle in the front center of the abdomen.

That, of course, is where we all seem to want a ton of muscle definition. And even though some of us realize that we can't spot reduce fat, they still insist on ignoring two-thirds of the muscles making up that all-important "ring" around the midsection.

Folks, the crunch is a fine exercise and it does its job well. But, there are a few other exercises we have to tack on to our abs routine to get the full effect.

First off, if there's a front, you know there's a back. The flip side of the coin when it comes to the six-pack are the erector spinae… the muscles of your low back. The six-pack muscles make you bend over at the middle, the erector spinae make you lean back in the opposite direction.

Then there's the sides. So that we don't get too involved in naming names, we'll just call them the obliques. They make you twist and bend to the side… and more importantly, support you in those directions as well.
The point is, you have a back and sides as well as a front, and to keep that ring of muscles strong enough to support your midsection like a weight belt, you have to work it all the way around. Remember that phrase, "a chain is only as strong as its weakest link"? You can't have any weak links if you want to protect your spine and support your internal organs.

Put another way, you wouldn't only build a fence across your front lawn and leave the sides and back yard open. What would that keep out? You have to fence the whole yard in.

From one thing, learn ten thousand things.

SCULPTING VS. BULKING

The next thing you need to understand when it comes to ab exercises is this: do NOT use heavy resistance.

A very simplified explanation goes like this. You have two kind of muscles… mover muscles and postural muscles. Mover muscles are designed to do just that… pick something up and move it, once. Well, once, or a couple of times.

Think of how we exercise our biceps. Pick up a heavy weight (large amount of resistance) and move it around eight or ten times (short duration of exercise). This promotes the increase in size that we're looking for, but not a lot of endurance.

That's a mover muscle. But that ring of muscle surrounding our midsection is a postural muscle; in other words, it supports a static position rather than moving an area.

Postural muscles keep us from collapsing, and they do that through a sustained contraction. Since there's no extra resistance involved, those postural muscles don't have to contract very hard, but they do have to sustain that contraction for a long period of time.

Mover muscles tend to be big and thick, but with little endurance (comparably). Postural muscles tend to be much smaller, but with excellent endurance (they'd better... they have to hold us up all day!)

The thing is, remember how adaptable our bodies are. Our tissues... be it bone, muscle, fat, whatever... will adapt to whatever kind of stresses they are exposed to, so long as they are not overwhelmed.

So if I start exercising a postural muscle (thin with endurance) like a mover muscle (thick with low endurance), what will happen?

It'll develop like a mover muscle. That means, "get bigger and thicker". Since most of us don't want a big thick abdomen... quite the opposite, in fact... we shouldn't exercise those muscles using heavy resistance.

Here's an example. Ever see one of those Olympic powerlifters, the ones that lift a really obnoxious amount of weight? Or my favorite, one of those Mega Man competitions on ESPN where huge guys are dragging trains and running with boulders and that sort of nonsense? Ever notice how they all have big round bellies?

It looks like a beer gut, but trust me, it isn't. If you gave that big round belly a punch, you'd hurt your hand.

That's because that big round belly is solid muscle. You see, those guys are putting so much stress on their midsection just to prevent collapsing under that heavy weight, that their abs and obliques and erector spinae have all hypertrophied (gotten bigger) to handle the added stress.

Those big abs don't need to support dragging a train or doing a five hundred pound squat for very long, but they do need to contract pretty darn hard to keep that competitor's spine from snapping.

Compare that to an Olympic swimmer. Not a big belly on that guy. In fact, his abs are much smaller and flatter than the powerlifter… but they have an incredible amount of endurance.

They have to… they're stabilizing the entire body for long stretches of swimming, during which the swimmer is creating constant torquing stress on the midsection by pulling and kicking with alternating arms and legs.

So…why, if you want a flat stomach like the swimmer, would you exercise those muscles with a plate loaded machine creating heavy resistance? That'll just bulk those abs up. You want to do exercises that offer a small amount of resistance, over a long time (or many repetitions).

HOW OFTEN/WHICH ONES?

When it comes time to actually setting up your abs training routine, here's how you're going to do it. It's really quite simple.

First, on any particular training day, make sure that you pick one exercise from each of the three areas of the midsection: Front, Side, and Rear abs. This will insure that you are training the entire "core" circle of muscles around your stomach.

Generally speaking, on each exercise, you're going to want to do it to "failure"; that is, keep doing repetitions of the exercise until you physically can't do them any longer. The nice thing about using light or no resistance (body weight) exercises is that it's easy for even a novice to get started. Hey, if you can only do one repetition… start with one.

Over time, of course, you will progress and get stronger, and therefore be able to do more repetitions.

How often should you train your abs? I would start with two days a week, and then add a third day after you stop getting sore all of the time a few days after training your abs.

You can eventually add another day and yet another until you're training abs five days a week, but work up to three for starters. Don't overwhelm yourself right out of the gate.

Besides, three days a week is enough for most people to achieve what they want.

CHAPTER 13:
EXERCISE: CARDIO TRAINING

Let's talk about cardiovascular training, usually called just "cardio", because we're all lazy and like to give things short nicknames. For most people, cardio is a love/hate relationship… you either love it, or hate it.

Love it or hate it, cardio is an important part of your training route. Like most of diet and exercise, how much cardio you do and what form it takes is really up to you and your particular goals.

It's also going to depend on your particular tastes. Do you prefer running? Hiking? Biking? Swimming?

Remember, the most important thing is that you do *something*. So don't be worried about "is biking better than running" or something like that. Get out there and *move*!

That being said, let's look at a couple basic principles of cardiovascular exercise.

HEART RATE AND INTENSITY

First off, we need to discuss a concept called *Maximal Heart Rate*. Maximal Heart Rate is, duh, the highest heart rate you can get, if you went all out and exerted yourself to the point of collapse.

Generally speaking, we don't directly measure maximal heart rate. We might hurt ourselves. So we typically estimate it, through a couple of different methods.

Why do we do this? To amuse ourselves, of course! Kidding, folks… it's because we're going to base our efforts and training on different percentages of that heart rate. But I'm skipping ahead.

The simplest way to estimate maximal heart rate involves an incredibly complex equation in which you subtract your age from 220. That's it. Once again, in case you missed it, that's 220 - AGE.

Tough, right? Of course, this is just an approximation, but the majority of people will have a maximal heart rate within 10 beats per minute of that number.

So what? you ask. *Why should I care?*

Good question. We use Maximal Heart Rate to figure out our exertion for cardio training, that's why. Generally speaking, you want to keep your heart rate during exercise between 60-80% of your maximal heart rate, depending on what you want to accomplish.

To focus your training on cardiovascular fitness (endurance) you want to keep your training in the higher end of that range (75-80%). If you want to focus on training your body to burn fat as fuel, stick to 60-70% MHR.

The most important factor in fat-burning, though, is the old calorie-in, calorie-out discussion we had a few chapters ago.

Always remember that you can't lose fat if you're taking in more calories than you're using.

YEAH, BUT WHO'S COUNTING?

Okay, so what if you're not too keen on constantly checking your pulse? I know I'm not. I feel a little silly jabbing a finger into my neck as I'm running, so I just use what's called *perceived exertion* to estimate my heart rate.

It's what it sounds like. You figure out how hard you're working, by how hard it *feels like* you're working. How do you rate your intensity from zero to ten, zero being I'm taking a nap, and ten being Good Lord, shoot me now!

Believe it or not, most of us can rate our exertion fairly accurately. The question is, what corresponds to what?

If you're classifying your exertion as "moderate" or slightly heavy… like a five or six on a ten point scale… you're probably in your fat-burning zone. If you're more like a seven or an eight, you're into endurance and cardiovascular fitness training. Above that, you're probably sprinting.

Of course, it couldn't hurt for you beginners to take your heart rate a couple of times in the beginning, just to see how accurate your perceptions are. Quite frankly, though, I think pulse rate is over-rated. Perceived exertion is quicker, easier, and just as accurate.

SURGE TRAINING FOR FASTER RESULTS

Another nifty tool you can use in your cardio training is called **surge training**. Simply put, surge training is training in high intensity bursts. You go heavy-duty for a bit, then you back off for a bit, then you go heavy duty again, and so on.

Think of this as an example. I'm running along the trail, do dee do, at a nice slow jog. Then I suddenly tear off at a sprint for a quarter mile. Then I slow back down to my nice slow jog. And so on.

That's surge training. Of course, it doesn't have to be done with running. You can do interval training on a bike, while swimming, whatever. The principle is the same.

The nice thing about interval training is, your heart rate will tend to stay fairly elevated even during your slow stretches. So, interval training can keep up a high heart rate while allowing you to change up your training a bit and avoiding a boring, plodding pace.

In addition, surge training is ideal for fat loss. A good rule of thumb is, go hard and fast for anywhere from one to five minutes, depending on your level of conditioning, and then back off until you get your breath back. Don't wait so long between intervals that you are fully rested; your heart rate should still be elevated.

THE IMPORTANCE OF CROSS TRAINING

The last topic I'll talk about when it comes to cardiovascular training is the importance of cross training. Cross training just refers to training that is outside of your normal routine; for example, if you're a runner, adding in biking or swimming from time to time.

Cross training has a number of benefits, the first of which is, not boring yourself to tears. Let's face it, we like a little variety in our lives, and running three miles yet again for the umpteenth time sometimes just doesn't cut it.

So, change it up. Strap on your swimming suit rather than your running shoes. Head out on your bike. Climb onto a rowing machine for a while.

The main benefit of cross training is **less injuries**. Most athletic injuries do not occur as the result of a one-time event; that is, we usually don't hurt ourselves by over-doing it for that last rep or running too hard on one occasion. It may seem that way, but that's not usually how it works.

The typical mechanism for injury is *repetitive micro-trauma*. Big words, which really just mean, doing the same thing the same way, over and over and over again until we wear our body (or at least a little chunk of it) down.

Our bodies can handle a tremendous amount of stress, but it needs time… and rest… to recuperate before the next stress hits. If we constantly beat down our bodies, every day, the same way in the same place, we can't rebuild what was broken down.

We don't break down right away, not noticeably. Nope, it's just a little, unnoticeable crack in the wall at first. But, if we keep going, and keep going, and keep going, hitting that same place in the same way over and over and over again, each little crack adds up, and gets larger, and bigger, slowly, until finally, the wall is weakened enough to breach under stress.

It isn't just in athletics that we find this. Occupational stresses are notorious for being repetitive. We sit at the same desk in the same way, tilting our head the same as always, all day, every day.

An hour like that won't hurt you. A day won't, either. But day after day, week after week, year after year, your body will break down by tiny degrees.

People are consistently shocked at how horrible their spinal X-rays look… until they realize they've been hunched over doing the same repetitive task for ten years. Then one day they bend over to tie their shoes. WHAMMO! Their low back locks up and now they can't stand up straight. It's classic.

It wasn't the shoe-tying that did it to them. It was the last fifteen years of contorting their bodies to fit pipes, or fix engines, or answer phones all day, or whatever their job required. It's an insidious, sneaky process, painless for years until finally we shock ourselves with a sudden, dramatic failure under stress.

Athletic injuries work the same way. Your body doesn't know it's exercising versus working versus anything else. It just reacts to stress according to natural law. Since the physical stresses of exercise tend to be greater than those encountered in our regular nine-to-five existence, the injuries are a bit accelerated, but they work the same way.

Overuse injuries are particularly common with cardiovascular work. Why? Well, because it is, by its very nature, more repetitive than resistance training. I might do three sets of ten repetitions of a bench press, that's thirty movements total. Compare that to how many times your little legs spin around to keep your bike moving forward for just ten minutes.

If I'm always running, running, running, you have the same impact… landing on your feet… over and over again, thousands of times in a row (well, maybe) each time you do it.

Is it any wonder that runners have problems with their knees or feet or hips or any number of other areas considering years of extremely repetitive stress? It should be a wonder that *more* people don't hurt themselves!

The point is this. If you change up the stresses on your body, you can continue to exercise with a much smaller chance of injury.

Yes, if I'm a competition runner, running is the best training for me, but by throwing in some swimming or other whatnot from time to time… *replacing* the running, not in addition to it… I can still work on increasing my endurance while not injuring myself.

Considering the time it takes to return from an injury, it's better to take this route than to push your limits and break your body down by little bits.

Since we're on the topic of pain and rest, let's go over that most misunderstood of pain, delayed onset muscle soreness.

DELAYED ONSET MUSCLE SORENESS

There's a lot of debate out there about delayed onset muscle soreness, which is a big fat term for getting sore after you exercise intensely for the first time in a while. In fact, some people seem quite concerned over this phenomenon, going to great lengths to figure out how to prevent it, treat it, avoid it, whatever. My personal feeling is, don't bother.

Remember that pain is the body's warning signal; our DON'T TOUCH or BETTER LOOK AT THIS sign. So let's take a look at what's happening when we get delayed onset muscle soreness.

First off, when do we get it? Exclusively after intense exercise, particularly when we're using muscles we haven't used in a while… in other words, muscles that are relatively weak. And it doesn't happen right away… it settles in the next day, and usually resolves within a day or two.

Is it a coincidence that this pain exists right where a tremendous amount of growth… muscle growth… just happens to be taking place? I doubt it. All of these people desperate to avoid delayed onset muscle soreness are missing the boat, in my opinion.

My best feeling is, delayed onset muscle soreness is a signal from our body, like all other pain, and in this case, the sign says DO NOT ENTER- UNDER CONSTRUCTION.

It's simple. When you exercise, you signal the body... through physical stress... that a particular area needs to be developed. So the body responds... ah, I'd better build that muscle up, it seems to be necessary... and begins rebuilding.

If rebuilding becomes a priority; as in, whoa, this weak little muscle that's been seriously underused now is suddenly being used, well, you wouldn't want anything to interfere with that, would you? So your body sends a signal... don't use this, I'm workin' here.

So what should you do about it? Nothing. And when I say "nothing", I don't just mean "don't change what you're doing", I mean, NOTHING. I do not advocate exercising on top of delayed onset muscle soreness.

 Quite the opposite. Your body is telling you to stay away from that area for a reason. It might be a positive reason... that we're building up muscle where there wasn't much to begin with... but it's still a reason.

 Now, you can probably exercise on top of very mild soreness without poor effect. But if you'd rate the soreness as being more than 1 on a scale of 1 to 10, then rest that area until the soreness subsides. If your chest is sore, exercise your legs. Otherwise, you're going to over-train your body, which can be just as bad as not training it, period.

EXERCISE DOESN'T BUILD MUSCLE...REST DOES!

Since we're on the topic, let's talk about rest in relation to exercise. Very often, I get people with the best of intentions come to me and ask, "Why aren't I getting stronger? I work out like crazy!"

That's their problem. So often, we get caught up in that "if a little of a thing is good, then a lot must be REALLY good!" mentality. Standing back from it, we observers can easily see the flaw in that logic.

Ha ha ha, we say. Silly person. Moderation is the key. But once you're in the middle of it, sometimes you need a neutral party to whap you over the head and tell you to knock it off.

Here's the thing about stress… a little is good, even necessary, but a lot overwhelms. Guys will hit the bench press like a wild devil, eight jillion sets a day, every day, and curse their horrible genetics since they can't seem to progress.

Or runners will put in eighteen miles of road work a day and wonder why they don't get faster (and keep getting injured). It's simple. They're overwhelming their bodies.

Elite athletes are usually aware of the secret behind real physical development; that exercise and training doesn't make you stronger or faster or whatever, it's your body's *response* to that exercise and training that makes you stronger and faster and whatever else you want to be.

That's a concept that's easy to nod your head to and say, "oh, okay," and at the same time really, really difficult to accept on a gut, emotional level. It doesn't seem to make sense. Rest doesn't make you strong, you say. Heck, I rest like it's my job; that's the problem. I rest so much it feels like my butt is turning to Jello.

The key is, it's not just rest. It's rest *following exertion*. The two are intertwined; have one, you get nothing, have both, you develop at an optimal rate.

I've been hammering on this point for a reason. Lots of people out there rush out and overwork themselves in the gym in a well-meaning, absolutely doomed attempt to speed their physical development along faster than is possible.

Change takes time, folks. Let it. We're impatient creatures that want it all now, now, now, but things just don't work that way. This is another reason why I advocate setting process goals rather than outcome goals. If I fixate on bench pressing three hundred pounds, I may tend to overwork myself in dogged pursuit of that goal and actually act in a counterproductive way.

So rest is important. The obvious question is, how much rest do you need?

Oh, I knew you'd ask that. The problem is, there's no easy answer to that. Each person's body is different, and their needs for rest are different. Even *more* fun, each person's needs for rest will change over time as they become more or less physically conditioned, or (remember our chapter on stress?) as life events increase or decrease the other sources of stress in that person's life.

Like everything else, you're just going to have to experiment with it. There's no spoon-feeding here. Go out and play with this. Take an active part in your own fitness.

It wouldn't hurt to consult with a personal trainer or other fitness expert. Very often, a third party observer can step back and see what little things we're doing to sabotage our own efforts… like not getting enough rest.

In the end, though, it's up to you to actually take control of your own life and your own body. Nobody else is going to do as good of a job as you, because nobody else has as much at stake as you. So don't just hand over your fitness and physique to somebody else. Dive in and play.

CHAPTER 14:
EXERCISE: RESISTANCE TRAINING

Resistance training has gotten a lot of press in the last decade or three, and for good reason… it has a ton of benefits and very few detractions. It's a vital part of any exercise habit; it's easy to ease yourself into, practically anybody can do it, and it fits perfectly into our method of using small stepping stones to form life-long patterns.

Let's start with listing some of the benefits. First off, there's the obvious… increase in muscle tone. Now, for those of you out there who are terrified of beginning any sort of weight lifting or other resistance training for fear of instantly transforming into a slightly smaller, less green version of the Incredible Hulk, let me evaporate those concerns for you.

The professional bodybuilders you see bulging their way up onto stage on ESPN spend two hours a day in the gym and eat every three or four hours (yes, some of them get up in the middle of the night just to eat) in order to look like that… and they do it for years and years to get into competition shape. It's highly unlikely you're going to bulk up like that with a mild to moderate resistance training routine.

On the other hand, an increase in muscle tone has dramatic health benefits. Less pain, for starters. More muscle development allows your body to maintain its structure against gravity or other physical stresses more easily… read that as helps to keep you from getting aches and pains like low back pain and other, similar maladies.

Your ligaments and tendons will also respond to resistance training by becoming stronger… so you become less likely to injure knees and elbows and all those other joints that are rather near and dear to us.

Bone density also increases as a result of resistance training. This is yet another example of the body's use-it-or-lose it attitude. Most people think of bones as dry, lifeless, brittle things that just kind of sit there like dumb rocks inside our bodies.

Nothing could be further from the truth. Bone is a vital, adaptable, living tissue with almost extraordinary properties. It responds to stress by building strength… read that as "density", the opposite of osteoporosis.

A GOOD DOUBLE WHAMMY

The big thing that we want from exercise, though, is weight loss. And, as we've discussed before, it's not really *weight* loss we want, but *fat* loss… so we can see those lovely muscles that we're shaping with exercise.

Remember when we calculated our BMR? That's the number of calories we burn just by being alive and sitting around on our butt. Well, one of the major components of how high your BMR clocks in at, is the amount of muscle tissue present in your body.

Muscle tissue burns up all kinds of energy just by being there; that's why we lose muscle when we're not using it. Your body doesn't want to waste energy on useless stuff.

What that means for you is, you get a double-whammy benefit from resistance training; not only does it burn up calories from the activity itself, but it also burns calories consistently throughout the day while you're doing nothing! Nice, hunh?

Let's take a look at an actual numerical example. Let's say you have a sedentary, 35 year old, 5'9" 170 pound man. His BMR would be 66 + (6.23x 170) + (12.7 X 69) – (6.8 X 35) or 1763. Multiplied by 1.2 for being sedentary, this person needs about 2,115 calories a day to maintain their weight.

Now we'll have that person gain ten pounds of muscle from weight training. Now his BMR is 66 + (6.23 X 180) + (12.7 X 69) – (6.8 X35) or 1825. Multiplied by 1.375 for what is now a light exercise lifestyle (we'll use light exercise just to be conservative) and now this same person needs 2,510 calories a day to maintain their weight.

Another way to look at this is, if this individual keeps their diet constant, those extra ten pounds of muscle will create a deficit of four hundred calories a day! This equates to a pound of fat about every nine days, or about three a month, or about thirty-five or forty pounds in a year.

Are we starting to see the benefits of resistance training yet?

BE A SHAPE-CHANGER

Another benefit of resistance training is that not only do you remove inches from where you typically don't want it, but you add inches where people tend to like to look. In women, the classic shape is referred to as "hourglass"; in men, we refer to the "V-shaped torso".

Whatever. We know it when we see it. And as I've mentioned before, some of us who aren't blessed with such a shape naturally can at least push ourselves in that direction with a little body sculpting.

Here's an example. Arnold Schwarzenegger. Yep, the Austrian Oak, seven-time Mr. Olympia, faked you out using this method. In his book, "Bodybuilding for Men", he mentions his tape measurements while in contest shape. His waist clocked in at 34 inches. While that might sound pretty good (and it is), compare it to Jack Lelane, the pioneer of American bodybuilding, who boasted a 28 inch waist.

The reason is, although Arnold's natural waist shape was a bit wider than his opponents'… even though the guy had practically zero fat on him… his *chest* size was a ridiculous 57 inches. Whoa! No wonder he won so many trophies!

Do you see what I'm talking about? He couldn't do anything more to make his waist actually smaller, so he made it look smaller by blowing his chest and back muscles up like an inflatable mattress. He also practiced posing a certain way to minimize attention to his waist, but that's straying off of the point.

The point is, even if we're not professional bodybuilders, we can still use the same tricks at our own level. I, too, am a bit narrow-challenged when it comes to the waist, so I make sure to keep my chest, back, and shoulders developed with resistance training so I edge a little closer to that "ideal" V-shape.

Remember, work with your body, not against it… and that counts with body shape as much as with our neurological patterns.

One of the quirks you'll discover as you begin resistance training is that some muscles will develop more quickly than others. It's important to recognize this and account for it in your training. Not just from an aesthetic point of view, either; tons of athletic injuries occur due to muscular imbalance.

As a personal example, the muscles of my limbs (shoulders, arms, and legs) tend to grow much more quickly and easily than those stuck to my torso (chest and back). I have to be careful not to do too much resistance training for my legs… if I did, they would balloon out in a ridiculously disproportionate manner compared to the rest of my body… not to mention my thighs rubbing together when I walk, which is annoying as well as uncomfortable.

SCULPTING VERSUS BULKING

As I mentioned before, the first concern most people have about resistance training is that it's going to make them "Huge", "muscle-bound", or some other synonym for grotesquely large. As I also mentioned before, that's pretty unlikely given the amount of time and effort required to get that big.

But, let's calm the nerves of those worried about busting out of their clothes overnight and go over the two basic ways to train with resistance… strength versus endurance.

When I say two basic ways, I really mean that as the two ends of a continuous spectrum. You don't really train for size or for endurance; any training provides both to some extent. We just favor one versus the other.

Strength training we'll define as **maximal effort training**… think of pushing up as heavy of a weight as you can, one time. By endurance, we really mean **localized muscle endurance**… like how many push-ups you can do before your arms turn into Jello and you fall flat on your face to the amusement of those of us watching you. Note that this is a little different from overall endurance, which is the kind we would associate with, say, a triathlete.

Strength training is typically associated with muscle size… the bigger the muscle, the more resistance it can handle. Local muscle endurance is a bit more complex, but it has to do with the efficiency of blood flow to that area and stuff like that.

Which is better? That depends. If you're interested in getting big, big, big, then you're going to favor heavy strength training. If you want muscle tone without getting too big, you're going to do much more local endurance-type work.

TERMS, TERMS, TERMS

To get more into the nitty-gritty of how and why this works, we need to define some stuff. Those of you familiar with resistance training will probably just skip over this part; those of you who don't know a super-set from a cantaloupe, read on.

We divide the discrete movements of each exercise into *sets* and *repetitions*. A repetition is the smallest unit, and just means doing the exercise one time, back and forth, up and down, whatever the movement is, you do it once. If we're doing push-ups, one repetition would be… you guessed it… lowering yourself down, and pushing yourself back up, one time.

A set is just a herd of repetitions. Any group of repetitions will do. If I do ten push-ups and then stop, that's a set. If I do fourteen sit-ups and then stop, that's a set.

You can get really tricky and mention how many repetitions or "reps" you did in each set… as in, "I did three sets of ten". If we're talking push-ups, that means you did ten push-ups, three times, with a little rest between each ten.

Pretty simple, right? We can get really wacky, and have a *circuit*, which is a series of exercises done right in a row with no rest in between, or a *superset*, which is two exercises for the same muscle group, done right in a row, or a *giant set*, which is three or four exercises for the same muscle group, done right in row. So if you did a bench press followed immediately by an incline press followed by pushups, this is a giant set, as those are all exercises for the chest.

This is different from a *circuit*, which is a series of exercises for the whole body. A *circuit* is usually done with a bit more rest between the exercises, and there might be ten exercises or more involved. The thirty-minute weight loss centers you see popping up all over the place typically rely on circuit training.

Another way of varying how you do your sets and reps is called a *pyramid*. That's when you do one set of an exercise with light weight and many reps, the next with heavier weight and less repetitions, the next with even heavier weight and even less repetitions, and so on. You can also go the other direction by starting heavy and ending light.

Some people like to focus on their *one rep max*. This is mostly for powerlifting and, to some extent, bragging, and is usually tested for the bench press, squat, and deadlift exercises.

It's what it sounds like. It's the maximum possible weight you can use to perform one repetition of a particular exercise. Think Olympic weightlifting competition.

One rep max is sometimes also used to help beginners figure out where to start. For example, if you want to start bench pressing, but you have no idea what weight to use, a personal trainer might test your one rep max for the bench press, and have you start at, say, eighty percent of that for six or eight repetitions. So it's not ALL about bragging rights.

The last term I'll fire at you is *failure*. Also what it sounds like. This is the point at which you just can't do one more repetition, no matter how hard you try. Generally speaking, you want to use enough weight and do enough repetitions so that you reach failure at the end of each set.

This is why it's important to have a *spotter*, or somebody watching you and assisting if necessary, so that you don't drop a heavy chunk of iron on your head after you reach failure.

There is value in hiring some professional help if you're a novice at exercise or even if you're just coming back from an, um, "extended hiatus". Personal trainers can put you on the right track, keep you on the right track, and most importantly, keep you from injuring yourself in front of that attractive person you've been eyeing up on the treadmill.

You can't learn karate by reading a book and looking at pictures. You have to have someone in white pajamas standing there, yelling at you while you're in a horse stance or something like that. Same thing. You could use some one on one, personal instruction on how to exercise properly if you really want to get results. You get what you give, remember?

Now that we know what we're talking about, what exactly should we do? How many sets, reps, whatever? Should we do circuits, super-sets, what?

As always, we want to determine what we're going to do by the goals that we've set. If our goals center around becoming a larger, more muscular version of ourselves, we're going to tend to work with heavier weights and less repetitions per set. If we're doing the local endurance dance, then we want more repetitions, with less weight.

When it comes to the number of sets we do per exercise, it's convenient to think of our body in terms of muscle groups. As we all know, not every action requires every single muscle in our body, and exercise is no different.

So we talk about working our legs, or chest, or back, arms, shoulders, and abdominal muscles (commonly now referred to as "the core" nowadays). Sometimes we split that up even more, like distinguishing working our biceps (front of the arm) from the triceps (back of the arm).

The basic muscle groups are broken down like this:

- Chest
- Back
- Arms
- Shoulders
- Legs

We're not going to go into the specific exercises for each body part and how to perform them… there just isn't room in this book. There are plenty of other books, magazines, and videos to show you all kinds of exercises… or better yet, enlist the aid of a nearby personal trainer.

Remember, you can't become a karate expert by reading a book on the subject; you need expert instruction from a professional. Learning to exercise works the same way.

Back in the old days, conventional wisdom was to train your entire body all in one day, three times a week. Nowadays, most exercise experts are suggesting that you not exercise a muscle group more than twice a week. Opinions vary, but most recommendations run something like this: exercise a body part once every four to seven days.

So, some people like to hit the aforementioned areas one at a time, one area a day, each day. This strategy has the benefit of allowing the exerciser to concentrate fully on that one part with maximal intensity.

Others prefer to "double-up" certain body parts so as to be able to hit them twice a week. Such a program might look like this:

Monday	Chest and Arms
Tuesday	Back and Shoulders
Wednesday	Legs
Thursday	Chest and Arms
Friday	Back and Shoulders

Again, this mostly boils down to personal preference. Should you exercise a muscle group once a week or twice a week? My answer is, "yes". Try each. See how it works for you. Or better yet, switch up from time to time, just to confuse yourself.

MACHINE VS. DUMBELL

Walk around any gym, and you'll see two distinct sections. One is full of exercise machines, and the other has piles of dumbbells and barbells with a couple of flat or angled benches; so-called "free weights". Depending on who you talk to, the debate can get pretty intense over which of the two you should favor.

So which do I recommend? As usual, my answer is, "yes".

Now, I'm not saying that just to be cute. The truth is, I can't know which you should use. That's because the answer depends on your individual situation. So let's look at the pros and cons of each so that you can make an informed decision.

First off, either one is better than nothing. Don't get so caught up in the idea that you have to use free weights that you won't ever, ever, ever use machines, or vice versa. That sounds pretty simple, but believe me, there's a lot of people out there who's preference for one or the other borders on fanaticism. Don't get caught in that trap.

Okay, so, here's the scoop on machines. Exercise machines are great because they're safe. Well, they're safe as long as you're using it properly, and not sitting backward or on your head or sticking your fingers in between the stacks of plates.

When using an exercise machine, your motion is restricted along a very certain track. This makes it extremely unlikely that your arm will suddenly go flying out at a strange angle if you get too tired.

So you're far less likely to injure yourself using a machine. This makes exercise machines ideal for beginners or people who are already injured and are in the initial phases of rehab.

Free weights, on the other hand, require the user to not only move the weight through the plane of motion for any given exercise, but also to stabilize that weight and keep it from flying off into the air and hitting some poor sod sitting nearby. This requires more effort and coordination. The exerciser has to engage secondary, stabilizing muscles to assist in the exercise.

Think of the difference between piloting a train versus an airplane. A train can only move along its track, forward or backward, so piloting it is relatively simple. An airplane, on the other hand, can move freely in any direction (once airborne) and so requires a lot more effort (and skill) to control.

So why use free weights? Because that extra effort seems to pay off. First off, people seem to build muscle more quickly with free weights than with machines. Also, since a free weight isn't locked into an artificially safer track of motion, training with free weights more closely resembles the true coordination of action of those muscles in a real-life, non-gym setting.

Hunh? you say. What I mean is this. Let's say I have to pick up a heavy bag of concrete off of the floor and put it onto a shelf over my head.

I think we'd all agree that in addition to the primary action of my legs and arms lifting the bag up into the air, I also have to *control* the motion of the bag, so that I don't drop it to the side, on my head, or topple over backwards onto an upturned rake.

With an exercise machine, the motion is locked into a track, so I don't have to worry about (or develop) my stabilizing muscles or coordination. But in the real world of using our muscles, there is no machine guarding our movements.

If you want to develop your body to handle real-life situations, you have to train it as such. This is particularly important for athletes; for them, coordination of their muscular effort is as important as the actual strength of the muscular contraction itself. It's not too hard to see how an extremely powerful contraction with little or no coordination can lead to injury.

Muscles are powerful, folks, more powerful than you think. You can contract a muscle hard enough to break a bone. I'm serious. I've seen it happen.

It's called an **avulsion fracture**, which is when the muscle contracts hard enough to jerk its tendon right off of its attachment to the bone. I saw a professor of mine give himself an avulsion fracture while playing baseball… he tried to steal third, and as he toed off to rush down the base line, he dropped screaming. He'd torn the base of his Achilles tendon off of his heel, with a little chunk of heel bone attached.

He didn't make the steal, by the way.

The point is, learning to control your muscular contraction (that's what coordination is) is as important, if not more so, than increasing the actual force of the contraction. This is where free weights shine.

So what's the down side? Well, since it's harder to control a free weight, it becomes easier to injure yourself if you don't know what you're doing. This is why I advocate working with a good personal trainer, at least at first.

Also, there's some muscles that you just can't reach the way you want to with free weights. You pretty much have to use some sort of machine, even if it's as simple as a chin-up bar.

Fantastic, you say. Great. But as usual, you've given us a big complex answer when all we wanted was a little simple one.

I know, I know. But remember, it's critical that you understand the principles behind how the machine we call the human body works. Then, you'll know what to do to reach your goals.

For those of you insisting on a short-cut, what I typically recommend is this. Use exercise machines if you're a beginner, if you're injured and starting your rehab, or if you have to use one to isolate a particular muscle. Otherwise, learn to use free weights and favor those.

Notice that I said injured people should *begin* on an exercise machine. It is my firm belief that an injured individual eventually must include real-life, non-machine exercises in their rehab program to regain as much utility as possible in the injured area. Your health care provider can give you more information.

PUTTING IT ALL TOGETHER

Remember how with our diet, we started off with one day a week, and so on and so forth, until we were up to six days a week of whole foods and one Cheat Day?

We'll do something similar with exercise. Except, exercise is a bit more variable, so we can actually be a bit more flexible with it.

Overall, the goal is to get to 3-5 days a week of each of the three kinds of training we've been talking about: abs training, cardio training, and resistance training.

The actual number will depend on you, your lifestyle, and your goals. More is better in this department, but you might not have the time to fit it all in.

Also, you may find you can fit some stuff in easier than others. If you love to run, you'll probably end up doing five days a week of cardio, and maybe less of the other exercise types.

That's okay. Just make sure you get in at least three days of both abs training and resistance training.

You can mix and match, too, depending on your schedule or even your whims. Three days a week of this one, four days of that, switch it around next week… whatever.

From time to time, even if you CAN do five days a week of each kind of training, you may want to back off for a while and give your body a bit of a rest. That's a great idea.

But for starters, just do ONE day of each. All on the same day, or spread out… I don't care. One day per week each of cardio, abs, and resistance training.

If and when that seems too easy, then go to two days a week of each. And then three, and so on, until you're up to that 3-5 days per week of each.

If you get overwhelmed, freak out, or just swamped with work and can't make all of your allotted training sessions in a week… relax. It's no big deal. Next week, you go right back to it.

If, on the other hand, you're getting overwhelmed consistently, you're progressing too fast. Back up a step. If you were overwhelmed at three days a week, go back to two until it feels too easy again. Then add that third day.

There's no law that says you have to progress in all three types of exercise at the same speed, either. If you jump up to three days a week of abs, two days of cardio, but are stuck at one for resistance training… then that's how it goes.

Again, this isn't a totalitarian regime. Go at the pace that works, so that you actually follow through. Done this way, it's a lot easier… and you'll see that it's really not such a big deal to exercise regularly after all!

Okay, my friends. At this point, you know more about diet and exercise than about 99% of the population, and about three-quarters of personal trainers.

Now you've got all the pieces of the puzzle: we've gone over the basics of diet and exercise that you need to know in order to lose the fat, AND more importantly, you've learned what you need to know about The Mental Game so that you can make that diet and exercise a consistent habit for a lifetime.

Chapter 15:
Summing It All Up

Let's summarize, now, everything we've covered so you can start your journey to dominating swimsuit season... not just this year, but EVERY year.

- Switch to a whole foods diet. Start by doing it just one or two days a week… depending on how bad your diet currently is… and add one more day a week **only when it becomes easy to do so**. The goal: Six days of whole foods, one Cheat Day.

- Add in a mix of cardio and resistance training to improve muscle tone, increase metabolism, and rapidly speed fat loss. Start with either one or two days of each, depending on your current exercise habits, and gradually add on more until you're doing 3-5 days per week of each type of exercise (depending on your schedule and just how much fat you want to lose).

- Train your abs three to five days a week as well, adding this training in the same way as cardio and resistance training. Be sure to exercise ALL parts of the abs; front, back, and sides.

- If you slip, cheat, stumble, or otherwise stray off of the path, don't freak out. Just shrug it off and get back on the path. You WILL have little hiccups along the way, due to stress or scheduling or other details of life.

Don't beat yourself up; just go back to improving your fitness habits step by step. If you get a flat tire, you don't give up and go home; you change the tire and get back on the road.

- Focus on the process, not the destination. It takes time to drive across the country, and it takes time to go from chubby to smoking hot. **Let it take time.** By focusing on your diet and exercise habits, you will insure that you will travel the path most efficiently and safely, and once you get into shape, you will STAY in shape.

- Don't get bogged down with chasing a lot of minor details of diet or exercise. Stick to getting the basics down, and doing the basics consistently. That's 99% of it. Tiny details like "should I do hammer curls or regular curls for my biceps?" are little more than a distraction.

- **FOCUS ON THE BIG THINGS**. Actually getting into the gym for 3-5 days each of cardio, resistance training, and abs training. Eating all whole foods, all the time, except for your cheat day. These are the things that will get you to where you want to be.

- And finally, have fun with it and be kind to yourself. This doesn't have to be a beating. In fact, it's better if it isn't. Enjoy the journey. Look around at the scenery. There is pleasure to be had in travelling this path.

You know now everything you need to know to get in the kind of shape you've always wanted to be in. And you know what path you need to walk in order to make it last for a lifetime.

Now it's time to actually walk that path.

Have fun, good luck, and I'll see you on the beach!

If you found this book helpful, be sure to check out my
website:

www.healthyandy.com

for more information on my nutritional supplements, books,
podcast, coupons and special offers, and free articles on all
kinds of stuff. I'm also on Twitter and Facebook under the
name Healthy Andy if you'd like to get some free health tips
sent to you.

www.ingramcontent.com/pod-product-compliance
Lightning Source LLC
Chambersburg PA
CBHW050908260726
48660CB00001B/100